Praise for
Reimagining Women's Cancers

"The illnesses of famous patients receive enormous attention from the media and serve as touchstones for patients and families dealing with similar conditions. They also can help vulnerable patients avoid being tricked by hoaxes, such as the unorthodox anticancer regimen that may have even accelerated Steve McQueen's death from mesothelioma. By taking a series of famous cancer cases and looking at the actual information being received by the public, Doctors Boguski and Berman are furthering the important process of ascertaining exactly what these episodes teach us."

—**Barron H. Lerner, MD, PhD,** Professor of Medicine and Population Health,
Division of Medical Ethics, New York University School of Medicine, New York
Langone Medical Center, author, *When Illness Goes Public:*
Celebrity Patients and How We Look at Medicine

"As an educator striving to effectively convey key points in a lecture, including a celebrity facet with other examples makes it easier for our students, trainees, and faculty to work through very complex concepts in a fun way. Celebrity Diagnosis provides credible information about health conditions and diagnoses for many popular figures today. I am able to use the resource in a professional capacity within the library as well in my courses and workshops on various topics related to genomic medicine and biomedical research."

—**Kristi L. Holmes, PhD,** Director, Galter Health Sciences Library
at Northwestern University, Feinberg School of Medicine

"You have demonstrated that the relationship between celebrity health conditions and consumer search behavior online has considerable potential for developing teachable moments for the advancement of public health. This is a highly innovative project with potentially big impact."

—**Nan M. Laird, PhD,** Harvey V. Fineberg
Professor of Biostatistics, Harvard School of Public Health

"Media coverage of celebrities contains little material that conveys useful health information. This is a missed opportunity that can and should be addressed."

—Dr. Katherine Smith, Johns Hopkins
Bloomberg School of Public Health

"*MedPage Today* found that since launching Celebrity Diagnosis on our site, page views have risen faster than any other blog we carry. We believe it's because celebrities attract attention as a jump-off point to educate. You have found a unique niche."

—Robert Stern, Advisory Board,
Everyday Health, former CEO, *MedPage Today*

"I must admit that using celebrity diagnoses as a platform for a book on cancer caught me off-guard, but then I read the manuscript—accurate, clear, useful information that the average person will read and understand, while realizing that some of their favorite celebrities have been through the same thing. If you or a loved one has been diagnosed with cancer or is at high risk, this book is for you."

—Ellen T. Matloff, MS, President and CEO
of MyGeneCounsel, founder and former director,
Cancer Genetic Counseling Program, Yale School of Medicine

Reimagining Women's Cancers

The Celebrity Diagnosis® Guide to Personalized Treatment and Prevention

Michele R. Berman, MD,
Mark S. Boguski, MD, PhD, FCAP,
and David Tabatsky

Health Communications, Inc.
Deerfield Beach, Florida

www.hcibooks.com

"I Am a Cancer Patient" by Amy Breitmann; "The Shower" by Laura L. Strebel; and
"Numbers to Live By" by Nisha Drummond.
From the book *Chicken Soup for the Soul: The Cancer Book*
by Jack Canfield, Mark Victor Hansen and David Tabatsky.
Copyright 2009 by Chicken Soup for the Soul Publishing, LLC.
Published by Chicken Soup for the Soul Publishing, LLC.

Chicken Soup for the Soul is a registered trademark of Chicken Soup for the Soul Publishing, LLC.
Reprinted by permission. All rights reserved.

"poem to my uterus" by Lucille Clifton from *Collected Poems of Lucille Clifton*.
Reprinted with permission of The Permissions Company, Inc.,
on behalf of BOA Editions, Ltd., *boaeditions.org*.

"Fried Gray Matter" by Claudia Carlson, © 2016 by Claudia Carlson (previously unpublished).

"I'm Becoming More Forgetful" by Jane Levin.
Reprinted with permission.

**Library of Congress Cataloging-in-Publication Data
is available through the Library of Congress**

© 2016 Michele R. Berman, MD, Mark S. Boguski, MD, PhD, FCAP, and David Tabatsky

ISBN-13: 978-07573-1953-2 (Paperback)
ISBN-10: 07573-1953-X (Paperback)
ISBN-13: 978-07573-1954-9 (ePub)
ISBN-10: 07573-1954-8 (ePub)

Publisher: Health Communications, Inc.
3201 S.W. 15th Street
Deerfield Beach, FL 33442–8190

Cover design by Larissa Hise Henoch
Interior design and formatting by Lawna Patterson Oldfield

Contents

Acknowledgments

We launched *CelebrityDiagnosis.com* in 2008 with a mission to provide a dynamic collection of Teachable Moments in Medicine® to increase health awareness and medical knowledge by reporting on common diseases affecting uncommon people and the lessons these cases can provide for all of us.

Early inspiration for this work came from Barron Lerner, MD, PhD, and his book, *When Illness Goes Public: Celebrity Patients and How We Look at Medicine*. We thank Dr. Lerner for his early encouragement and continuing support.

Two other early supporters were Robert Stern, former CEO of *MedPage Today*, who first brought our work to the attention of healthcare professionals, and Helen Osborne, author of *Health Literacy from A To Z: Practical Ways to Communicate Your Health Message*, who increased awareness of our work through her *Health Literacy Out Loud* podcasts.

When Dr. Nan Laird of the Harvard T. H. Chan School of Public Health learned about our venture into celebrity health journalism, she initially counseled us to keep our day jobs. We thank her for advice and steadfast support, particularly in applying for grant funding from NIH.

Kirsten Ostherr, PhD, MPH, recognized the unique pedagogical value of our work and incorporated it into her popular course on *Medicine & Media* at Rice University. We thank Professor Ostherr and her students for their contributions to our mission.

Joel Aronowitz, MD, of the Breast Preservation Foundation, and Stephanie Holvick, RN, of *RNFaces.com*, educated us about the aesthetic and psychological dimensions of treating and recovering from cancer. We thank them for allowing us to interview them for our book.

Michael Misialek, MD, at Newton-Wellesley Hospital, Ellen Matloff, MS, CGC, at *MyGeneCounsel.com*, and Georgia Hurst, at *www.IhaveLynchSyndrome.com*, expended considerable time and effort in reviewing the medical content of our book and for this we are very grateful. Although every effort has been made to ensure that the information was correct and up to date at press time, any errors or omissions are the responsibility of the authors.

Margaret Foti, PhD, MD, (hc) of the American Association for Cancer Research has been a friend and colleague for more than twenty years. We share a passion for educating people about cancer and we thank her for her continuing friendship and sponsorship of our work.

Dr. Paul Laffer has been a valued adviser and enthusiastic supporter of our mission.

And, of course, we are grateful to Nancy Rosenfeld, our literary agent, for connecting us with HCI; Christine Belleris, Kim Weiss, and the entire team have been great to work with and we look forward to continuing our relationship with them as this series evolves.

We would be remiss not to acknowledge the celebrities included in this book who have made their stories available to the general public. Their willingness to help create these Teachable Moments in Medicine cannot be underestimated. We encourage other celebrities to also come forward and share their stories, as they play valuable roles in educating the public and inspiring them to take whatever preventative measures they can in maintaining good health.

David Tabatsky has been a phenomenal partner in this endeavor. His skill and experience are only matched by his warmth and humanity, and this project simply wouldn't have been possible without him. Thank you, David!

The final stages of book production competed for our attention with preparations for our daughter's wedding. We were able to pull off both by heeding Wilfred Arian Peterson's advice in *The Art of a Good Marriage*, including being flexible, patient, understanding and having a sense of humor.

—Michele Berman and Mark Boguski
Boston, MA

I would like to thank Michele and Mark for their lovely dispositions, friendship, and clearheaded approach to such a complicated subject. It's a total pleasure to work with them.

I'd also like to thank Nancy Rosenfeld, Christine Belleris and everyone at HCI for their commitment to this project.

Finally, may I acknowledge the wonderful people who have inspired the *My Journey* stories in both of these books. You inspire more people than you could ever imagine.

And to Dani, Bob, Jamie, Jan, Linn, and Rick—my love and gratitude.

—David Tabatsky
New York City

Introduction

Information is empowering, especially when it's dispensed in manageable doses. Reading about people coping with cancer—the same one you are dealing with—is not only educational and inspiring, it can save a life. Couple that with our fascination with celebrities and there is much we can learn from their experiences.

Celebrity cancer memoirs, including *The Time of My Life* by Patrick Swayze and Lisa Niemi Swayze (Atria 2010), *Resilience: Reflections on the Burdens and Gifts of Facing Life's Adversities* by Elizabeth Edwards (Broadway Books 2006), *Cancer Schmancer* by Fran Drescher (Grand Central Publishing 2002), *Time on Fire: My Comedy of Terrors* by Evan Handler (Little, Brown and Co. 1996, Argo-Navis 2012), provide readers with a behind-the-scenes look at how a famous person dealt with a cancer challenge that may be common to many of us. Not surprisingly, their struggles are essentially no different from any of ours.

It's no secret that celebrity information not only sells, it can educate people about many important issues—including cancer.

According to *USA Today*, when Katie Couric's colonoscopy was broadcast on live television, colonoscopy rates rose more than 20 percent. When Michael Douglas shared his throat cancer story, he taught us about the connection between human papillomavirus (HPV), oral sex, and head and neck cancers. Angelina Jolie's op-ed in the *New York Times*, detailing her genetic predisposition to breast and ovarian cancers, and her subsequent decision to undergo a bilateral mastectomy, educated millions of people on the issue of genetic screening and preventative treatments and inspired them to take a proactive role in managing their own health.

Hamish Pringle, author of *Celebrity Sells* (John Wiley & Sons 2004) and former Director General of the Institute of Practitioners in Advertising, explains that "the role celebrities play in people's lives goes beyond a voyeuristic form of entertainment; they actually fulfill an extremely important research and development function for them as individuals and for society at large. People use celebrities as role models and guides."

That's what "infotainment" can do and what we hope *Reimagining Women's Cancers* exemplifies by dedicating itself to specific cancers affecting women and the people they love.

Because every twenty-three seconds someone in America is diagnosed with cancer, the number of people affected is continuing to grow and the data is not encouraging. The American Cancer Society estimates that nearly 2 million *new* patients will need treatment in the coming year. A recent World Cancer Report from the World Health Organization expects a 57 percent rise in cancer cases in the next twenty years.

Christopher Wild, director of the International Agency for Research on Cancer, says, "We cannot treat our way out of the cancer problem. More commitment to prevention and early detection is desperately needed in order to complement improved treatments and address the alarming rise in the cancer burden globally."

The report says about half of all cancers are preventable and can be avoided if current medical knowledge is better delivered. The disease could be tackled by addressing lifestyle factors, such as smoking, alcohol consumption, diet, and exercise; adopting screening programs; or, in the case of infection-triggered cancers such as cervical and liver cancers, through vaccines. "The rise of cancer is a major obstacle to human development and well-being," Wild says. "Immediate action is needed to confront this human disaster."

This emphasis on prevention and early detection demonstrates the necessity and value of education. It is the key for anyone who might otherwise not pay attention to an epidemic that is likely to affect him or her or a loved one.

But a diagnosis of cancer is not—and does not have to be—an automatic death sentence. With advances in genomic (DNA) testing and diagnosis, we have learned that cancer—if detected early—can be managed just like many other chronic diseases or, in many cases, prevented through changes in diet, exercise, and general lifestyle.

That includes developing a sense of humor, which has proven time and time again to help everyone, from patients to doctors and especially those who can't figure out what to do or say when confronted with such a big challenge.

Consider the story of Allison from upstate New York, who grew used to people staring at her bald head. One day a stranger nearly stalked her in a grocery store until she stopped her for what seemed to be a "classified" question, asked in a sympathetic whisper, as if no one else should know. "Did you lose your hair?" the woman said.

Allison smiled. "Lose my hair?" she said. "Oh, no. It's just invisible."

The stranger stared at her in shock. Then she started to giggle, and so did Allison, who wished her a good day and continued on with her shopping.

Actress and breast cancer survivor Christina Applegate told *womens healthmag.com* in 2013, "I laughed more in the hospital than I ever have in my life, making fun of all the weird things that were happening to me. My friends would walk in with this sad look, and I would throw something at them and say, 'Come on! This isn't the end of the world!'"

This book is full of anecdotal evidence—from celebrities we have come to admire and trust as well as from "normal" people with valuable viewpoints of their own who together offer us remarkably useful teachable moments that can educate and inspire and, in some cases, serve as life-saving cautionary tales.

Celebrity Diagnosis, the website we founded and launched in 2009, which is now featured as an integral part of the American Association for Cancer Research (AACR) Foundation website, combines celebrity health conditions (diagnosis, treatment, survivorship, etc.) with up-to-date medical information on common and uncommon cancers. By doing so, we have created numerous teachable moments in medicine, leading visitors to increase their health awareness and medical knowledge, which subsequently increases the likelihood of their considering early detection and preventative behavior.

"We have found from our own reporting on medical news," says Robert Stern, CEO of *MedPage Today*, a leading source of medical information online, "that nothing resonates with our professional clinician readers more than a celebrity illness because call volume to offices increases from patients when a celebrity is diagnosed. This provides a teachable moment for the physician to share with the patient."

The AACR, with its 35,000 members from around the globe, making it the oldest and largest scientific organization in the world, agrees, and by featuring Celebrity Diagnosis it is now expanding its support of high-quality, innovative cancer research and education. Through its numerous publications and frequent conferences, the AACR works with a vast umbrella of cancer organizations, hospitals, and individuals.

Meanwhile, the pharmaceutical industry, with its mission to address unmet medical needs by developing new drugs, still takes ten to fifteen years at an average cost of $1 billion to sponsor the applied research, tech development, and organizational structure to develop a single new drug, which may or may not serve its intended purpose.

What about the needs of consumers for better access to existing medical knowledge and practices? Can increasing health awareness and providing scientific information lead to better use of existing resources, including prevention and early detection screening methods? Social media and mass market books can be valuable allies in the task to equip people with what is necessary to manage and improve their own health.

We certainly hope so. That's why our philosophy of Participatory Medicine is a lynchpin of Celebrity Diagnosis and a key to empowering people to partner with their doctors in taking responsibility for their healing.

The definition of a modern "e-patient" is to be *engaged, equipped,* and *empowered,* three integral qualities that form the foundation of our approach.

Dr. Katherine Smith of Johns Hopkins Bloomberg School of Public Health feels that traditional media coverage of celebrities contains little material that conveys useful health information, concluding that, "media attention to such newsworthy events is a missed opportunity that can and should be addressed."

We agree. There seems to be a large missed opportunity to educate people about prevention and personal empowerment. That's why *Reimagining Women's Cancers* now exists—to inform, inspire, and ignite the appropriate type of action that is needed to live healthier lives. But you may ask, what does a famous person have to do with me?

Studies of the power of celebrity to create teachable moments, such as those conducted by Professor Graeme Turner of the University of Queensland Centre for Critical and Cultural Studies, Hamish Pringle at the Institute of Practitioners of Advertising, and Robert Havighurst, PhD, author of *Human Development and Education,* suggest that the personal life experiences of individuals we admire and respect from popular culture can create teachable moments that may be vicarious at first but ultimately prove to be educational and, in some cases, lifesaving.

According to Mable Kinzie of the University of Virginia Curry School of Education, who has developed instructional design strategies for health behavior change, there is a five-step process to developing educational materials that resonate and connect, producing real results.

It begins with gaining attention by featuring famous people whose health has become a news item, and then providing information on specific conditions (in this case, women's cancers). It continues by offering guidance through clear and concise information about how a particular cancer exists and operates, as well as anecdotal reports, interviews, and expert medical resources. When presented together, these enhance retention and stimulate appropriate social discourse that inevitably shares this knowledge with others.

For someone newly diagnosed with breast, ovarian, endometrial/ uterine, or cervical cancers—or for those suddenly thrust into the role of caregiver—the medical information provided here is easy to find and read, providing you with a comprehensive overview of the particular cancer's traits, warning signs, symptoms, diagnostic techniques, as well as prognoses and treatments, both traditional and alternative. This medical information is complemented by personal accounts and interviews from celebrities and non-celebrities who have been challenged by the same cancers.

For example, the chapter on breast cancer begins with a view of basic anatomy; an overview of how we view breast cancer today; signs, symptoms, and diagnosis; as well as scientific information on mammogram guidelines and ultrasound. You'll find a comprehensive survey of treatments, breast reconstruction, prevention, and short- and long-term forecasts.

Woven throughout the book are celebrity stories, both medical and anecdotal, from women including Angelina Jolie, Joan Lunden, Melissa Etheridge, Sandra Lee, Rita Wilson, Christina Applegate, and Suzanne Somers, as well as stories from women you may recognize as neighbors, colleagues, and friends.

Since scientific concepts such as DNA and the human genome have become commonplace through television shows like *CSI* and *Dr. Oz*, as well as in other media like the *New York Times* and *Time* magazine, this vital information is now more accessible than ever and much better understood by the general public, enabling patients and caregivers to raise their level of interaction with their doctors.

We like to cite the Angelina Jolie Effect, which has caused curiosity about cancer and DNA/genetic testing to skyrocket, as more and more patients are asking to have their tumor genomes analyzed in order to select the right drug treatment for them.

When news of a celebrity being diagnosed with cancer goes public, physicians invariably see a sharp increase in the volume of calls to their offices, and online search-engine traffic spikes for the specific disease or medical condition associated with that celebrity diagnosis. We refer to this interface between health communication and pop culture as the Goody-Gaga Effect, which refers to the sharp increase in public interest in a specific disease or medical conditions when it is associated with a celebrity. The Goody-Gaga Effect is named after the late British TV personality Jade Goody, whose battle with cervical cancer was followed daily in the UK, and Lady Gaga, who made her "borderline positive" lupus test public, prompting a huge spike in the attention and support given to that disease.

But when celebrities (or their publicists) talk about cancer or other medical issues, the results can be mixed. If they mistakenly publicize information that is confusing or contradictory to established medical protocols, they may cause harm. On the other hand, when they provide the public with an accurate, inside look at their situation, this can become a teachable moment and lives can be saved. Exploring examples of how this works is not only instructive and, in some cases, entertaining, it colors the way we essentially view celebrity and the manners in which we might disseminate and digest life-altering information.

Brian L. Dyak, president and cofounder of the Entertainment Industries Council and the Entertainment and Media Communication Institute and the award-winning creator of the PRISM Awards (FX Networks) television special, is a pioneer of "edutainment," which promotes the power of celebrity to depict health issues. For over twenty-five years, Dyak has successfully constructed a bridge between the entertainment industry and health and social policy issues. His thoughts on the link between the entertainment industry and national health have inspired us to reach more people with the foundational information you will find in this book.

Unfortunately, cancer is not going away anytime soon but neither is our fascination with celebrities, especially when they—like any of us—become vulnerable. With this in mind, the need to educate and heal is clear. For the more than 354,000 women who are diagnosed with cancer each year in the United States—as well as for the loved ones and medical professionals who care for them—we hope this book will offer great benefits.

Barron Lerner, MD, Professor of Medicine and Public Health at Columbia University College of Physicians and Surgeons, demonstrates in his book *When Illness Goes Public: Celebrity Patients and How We Look at Medicine* how celebrities significantly influence public attitudes toward diseases and their treatments. Lerner concludes that celebrity cases can educate the public, create advocates for research and care on behalf of other people with the same disease, and even influence aspects of the professional training of physicians.

By exercising the powerful magic of storytelling, celebrities are capable of influencing people in a wide variety of ways. But they can do much more than move us emotionally. They can raise our awareness about cancer and, in many cases, even prompt their fans to become better informed and seek the preventative care and early diagnostic screening they need.

People in the public eye have the potential to provide teachable moments in medicine. We can learn from them, as we can from nearly anyone who has experienced cancer as a patient or caregiver. They all have wisdom to share. And medical professionals of all stripes have much insight to offer.

Together, the anecdotes and experiences shared here in *Reimagining Women's Cancers* provide a substantial collection of cancer portraits, and, along with all of the comprehensive medical information, you should be able to find much of what you may need in order to understand what you are dealing with and to figure out how best to proceed. Most important, you will be better equipped to communicate effectively with your doctors, which should provide you the best-case scenario for making what can often be difficult choices.

Emmarie Truman, who was diagnosed with cancer as a teenager, was given a button one day while in a radiation room that read Cancer Sucks. She agreed that this is the best way to look at it. "Cancer does suck," she said, "and the sooner you accept that, the sooner you can realize that no matter how much it sucks you have to deal with it, and that you might as well deal with it with a smile."[1]

This simple lesson is not one to be overlooked. You will find that *Reimagining Women's Cancers* is full of them. By combining the inspiration of "average" patients and the power of celebrity stories with vital information about common and uncommon cancers, we hope that this book will help you become better informed as a patient and/or patient advocate.

In his State of the Union address earlier this year, President Obama announced a new Moonshot to Cure Cancer campaign, which follows the Precision Medicine Initiative launched a year earlier—both inspired, in part, by the tragic loss of Vice President Joe Biden's son Beau to cancer in 2015. Such a high-profile case can lead to increased awareness in the general public, as well as launch renewed efforts on governmental and private institutional levels to prevent and eventually eradicate this disease.

In the chapters that follow, we'll explain why the time is ripe, as MD Anderson Cancer Center says, to "make cancer history" through

---

1. From *The Cancer Book: 101 Stories of Courage, Support & Love* (Chicken Soup for the Soul Publishing, 2009).

the cutting-edge practice of precision medicine using sophisticated, targeted treatments that attack the root causes of the disease.

Together, we can make a difference.

A Note on Resources and Celebrity Diagnosis

Throughout *Reimagining Women's Cancers*, we present relevant scientific data about each type of cancer discussed in a particular chapter. Because this book is not primarily intended to be a textbook for medical students/doctors but rather a guide and teaching tool for *anyone*, we have attempted to dose out the medical information in easy-to-read and appropriately digestible pieces that will be manageable and satisfying.

Those seeking additional medical information/anecdotal stories about other celebrities with cancer can visit either of our companion websites: *www.celebritydiagnosis.com*; *www.reimaginingcancer.com*.

A Note on Non-Celebrity Stories

In an effort to provide as comprehensive a collection as possible of patients and caregivers affected by women's cancers, we have selected from a wide assortment of anecdotes, blogs, interviews, and stories from women and men throughout the country.

Each of the My Journey segments you will come across represents an individualized composite of the many people we have been in contact with over the past several years. In some cases the names have been changed to protect their privacy.

1

A NEW MIND-SET:
Reimagining Cancer
as a Manageable
Chronic Illness

The only person who can save you is you:
That was going to be the thing that
informed the rest of my life.

—Sheryl Crow, as told to *Reader's Digest*

The Evolution of Cancer Treatment:
From Toxic "Weapons of Mass Destruction"
to Targeted Therapy

Alexa Score is a twenty-six-year-old elite professional wakeboarder. In 2006, she began experiencing frequent hot flashes and night sweats. Doctors found her blood clogged with white cells containing something called the Philadelphia chromosome, and the diagnosis was a type of leukemia called CML. This threw Alexa's plans of being a normal teenager for a serious loop.

But if she had been diagnosed with CML ten years earlier, in 1996, the next steps would have been a series of injections with toxic drugs, similar in its chemical composition to mustard gas, a World War I–era weapon of mass destruction, followed by irradiation of her entire body.

These treatments were meant to destroy DNA and the cancer cells along with it. But since DNA is present in all human cells, the chemotherapy and radiation couldn't discriminate between cancer and normal cells. That is why this type of therapy is plagued by toxic side effects. Many types of cancer, not just CML, were, and still are, treated with these chemicals and radiation, which we often refer to as weapons of mass destruction (WMDs).

So what changed the landscape in those ten years? It was the introduction in 2001 of Gleevec, the first "magic bullet" cancer drug. Instead of offering treatment with a WMD cocktail, the twenty-first century war on cancer is now conducted with the medical equivalent of precision-guided smart munitions, similar in concept to smart bombs and precision-guided missiles. All of these weapons are designed to specifically target cancer cells and minimize collateral damage.

Alexa Score and the Magic Cancer Bullet

Alexa received treatment with one of these targeted therapies—a little orange pill called imatinib, known commercially as Gleevec. These "magic cancer bullets" have now become the gold standard for treatment of CML and many other types of cancer, including skin (melanoma) and lung cancers. Approximately three dozen additional targeted therapies, similar to imatinib, are now approved by the U.S. Food and Drug Administration (FDA). Hundreds more are in development by drug companies.

According to the FDA, imatinib is now used to treat several types of leukemia and other cancers of the bone marrow. It is also used to treat gastrointestinal stromal tumors and a rare sarcoma.

The lesson of Gleevec is that once we understand the underlying cause of a cancer and can precisely diagnose it, this knowledge almost always extends to other cancers as well.

Dr. Francis Collins and Christopher Hitchens: The Language of God Meets Personalized Medicine

Dr. Francis Collins was the director of the Human Genome Project and is the current director of the National Institutes of Health (NIH). Dr. Collins is also an evangelical Christian who wrote a book about DNA, defining genes as *The Language of God*.

Dr. Collins often engaged in friendly debates about God's existence with author, journalist, and celebrated atheist Christopher Hitchens. When the sixty-year-old Mr. Hitchens was diagnosed with cancer of the esophagus in 2010, Dr. Collins reached out to his debate partner with the possibility of using advanced DNA techniques to analyze Hitchens's cancer and pick the right treatment, a process sometimes called personalized medicine.

While Hitchins was not suffering from a gender specific cancer, his story is instructive. The standard treatment for cancer of the esophagus is surgery, but Mr. Hitchens's cancer had already spread and was in its most advanced state: stage IV. As Mr. Hitchens dryly observed, "There is no stage V." For Mr. Hitchens's advanced cancer, the treatment was similar to what a CML patient would have received in 1998—chemical and radiation WMDs.

But Dr. Collins and his colleagues made a startling discovery in Hitchens's tumor's DNA. They identified a "misprint" that might respond to the same drug that turned Alexa Score's cancer into a manageable chronic illness: imatinib.

Today, in an increasing number of cases, cancer is being transformed from a deadly disease into a manageable chronic illness. This reimagining of cancer is made possible by research advances that allow more precise diagnosis and personalized treatment. New technologies are emerging (Chapter 14) that will enable detection and diagnosis of cancer in a drop of blood rather than in a piece of the cancer surgically removed from a patient.

MY JOURNEY

I got diagnosed on a Thursday and faced a long weekend with the news before my next appointment on Monday. I spent most of that time stuck in my head, freaking out, and searching online for cures. When I returned to the doctor, she explained a whole bunch of stuff that sounded like a foreign language, and then she asked me if I had any questions. I felt like a failure because I didn't have anything written down and basically no other thoughts in my head besides "Am I going to live?" I couldn't think straight and went home feeling very frustrated and afraid.

Amelie (Burlington, Vermont)

Crucial Questions for Your Doctor

For the more than 350,000 women who are diagnosed each year with new cases of breast, ovarian, fallopian, uterus, cervix, vulvar, and vaginal cancers, there are a host of crucial questions they should ask their doctor. Our friends at *www.surviveit.org* suggest these questions:

- Exactly what type of cancer do I have?
- What stage is my cancer in, and does that affect my options?
- Is there any further testing available to better diagnose my cancer?
- Was my biopsy analyzed for any specific gene mutation(s)?

- Can further gene mutation testing diagnose my cancer more specifically?
- If the gene mutation testing is negative, what treatment options are available?
- Should I see a certified genetic counselor to determine if my cancer is hereditary?
- What do you recommend and why, and where can I learn more about this type of treatment?
- What risks or side effects are there to the treatment(s) you suggest?
- How is the treatment likely to help, and when will we know if it's working?
- What is the five-year survival rate for my specific condition?
- Can you put me in contact with someone you treated with this treatment plan?
- Are there any clinical trials I should consider?
- Who is researching my type of cancer, and should I seek a second opinion from them?
- If they offer a targeted treatment plan or clinical trial, will you collaborate with them?
- How do you recommend I share my hopes and expectations with my family?
- What should I do to be ready for my next phase of treatment?

Once you've asked these questions, hopefully your doctors, nurses, and social workers will be asking appropriate questions of you. After all, they are human, too, and dealing with patients full time can be a humbling reminder of their own fragility.

"Those of us who work in oncology make a pact with the gods," says Hester Hill Schnipper, LICSW, BCD, OSW-C, chief of oncology social work at Beth Israel Deaconess Medical Center in Boston. "If we devote our lives to taking care of others, our own lives, and those of people whom we love, will be protected. Intellectually, we know that it's not so, but in our hearts, the contract is sealed."

The effects of cancer challenge the humanity of patients *and* medical professionals. That's why effective communication in both directions is essential to everyone's good health.

─────────────── MY JOURNEY ───────────────

After being diagnosed and working out a treatment plan with my oncologist, I went to buy the medicine I'd been prescribed. I was trying to pretend that it was just like getting an antibiotic for a normal infection. But my pharmacist recognized my anxiety and gave me some wise advice.

"One of the most important things to remember in the months ahead is what's between your ears," he said. "Your mind-set will play a big part in how you deal with this whole process."

I couldn't thank him enough. Between my doctor's positivity and my pharmacist's spelling out for me the importance of maintaining a positive attitude, I've been constantly reminded to be grateful for each day and the people who make them valuable.

Taylor (Columbus, Ohio)

The Basics: Grading and Staging Cancer

Two terms we often hear when a doctor speaks about cancer are its *grade* and *stage*. "What grade is your cancer?" and "What stage is it?" are questions often asked of a patient or his or her loved one.

Just when you thought you might be done being evaluated as a person, when your school days were a distant memory in your rearview mirror, the scientific facts of a cancer diagnosis can sling-shot you back to those days of being graded and placed on a level of someone else's ladder. So, like nearly any other new challenge you may face in life, it's essential that you know the landscape and find out where you stand.

Grade is a term used in the study of pathology. When a pathologist looks at cancer cells under a microscope, he or she determines its grade. How close a cancer cell resembles the kind of cell from which it originates will determine its grade.

Stage, a term referring to a particular cancer's stage, is based on how deeply a tumor has invaded its originating organ and whether it has spread locally or distantly from its original site.

What Is a Tumor Grade?

Tumor grade is the description of a tumor based on how abnormal the tumor cells and the tumor tissue look under a microscope. It is an indicator of how quickly a tumor is likely to grow and spread. If the cells of the tumor and the organization of the tumor's tissue are close to those of normal cells and tissue, the tumor is called "well differen-tiated." These tumors tend to grow and spread at a slower rate than tumors that are "undifferentiated" or "poorly differentiated," which have abnormal-looking cells and may lack normal tissue structures.

Based on these and other differences in microscopic appearance, doctors assign a numerical grade to most cancers. The factors used to determine a tumor's grade can vary between different types of cancer. Let's examine how a tumor grade is determined.

If a tumor is suspected to be malignant, a doctor removes all or part of it during a procedure called a biopsy. A pathologist—a doctor who identifies diseases by studying cells and tissues under a microscope—then examines the biopsied tissue to determine whether the tumor is benign, meaning without any sign of cancer and usually not harmful, or malignant, which usually indicates something severe and serious, especially if it grows or spreads.

The pathologist also determines the tumor's grade and identifies other characteristics of the tumor, such as its origin, structure, rate of growth, and level of invasiveness.

You might be asking, how are tumor grades classified?

Grading systems differ depending on the type of cancer. In general, tumors are graded as 1, 2, 3, or 4, depending on the amount of abnormality.

In grade 1 tumors, the tumor cells and the organization of the tumor tissue appear close to normal. These tumors tend to grow and spread slowly.

In contrast, the cells and tissue of grade 3 and grade 4 tumors do not look like normal cells and tissue. Grade 3 and grade 4 tumors tend to grow rapidly and spread faster than tumors with a lower grade.

If a grading system for a tumor type is not specified, the following system is generally used to identify a tumor's grade:

- *GX:* Grade cannot be assessed (undetermined grade)
- *G1:* Well differentiated (low grade)
- *G2:* Moderately differentiated (intermediate grade)
- *G3:* Poorly differentiated (high grade)
- *G4:* Undifferentiated (high grade)

Grades and Treatment

A tumor's grade always affects a patient's treatment options. It begins with how doctors use that specific information and other factors, such as a cancer's stage and a patient's age and general health, to develop a treatment plan and to determine a patient's prognosis—the likely outcome or course of a disease, that is, the chance of recovery or recurrence.

Generally, a lower grade indicates a better prognosis. A higher-grade cancer may grow and spread more quickly and may require immediate or more aggressive treatment.

The importance of tumor grade in planning treatment and determining a patient's prognosis is greater for certain types of cancer, such as soft tissue sarcoma, primary brain tumors, and breast and prostate cancer.

Staging

This term describes the extent or severity of an individual's cancer and is based on the size and scope of the original (primary) tumor, as well as if and how it has spread in the body, and to what degree. This is important for a few reasons.

- It helps the doctor plan a person's treatment.
- It can be used to estimate the person's prognosis.
- It can help identify clinical trials (research studies) suitable for a particular patient.

Staging helps researchers and healthcare providers exchange information about patients. It also gives them a common language for evaluating the results of clinical trials and comparing the results of different trials. It will be helpful to define the five stages of cancer.

- *Stage 0:* Carcinoma *in situ* (early cancer present only in layer of cells in which it began).
- *Stages I/II/III:* Indicates more extensive disease, greater tumor size/spread of the cancer to nearby lymph nodes/organs adjacent to the primary tumor.
- *Stage IV:* The cancer has spread to another organ.

Tumors and Systems

Staging is based on an acquired knowledge of the way cancer develops. This usually begins with defining a cancerous tumor. Cancer cells divide and grow without control or order, which eventually form a mass of tissue called a growth or tumor. As the tumor grows, it can invade nearby organs and tissues. Cancer cells can also break away from the tumor and enter the bloodstream or lymphatic system. When this occurs, cancer can spread from the primary site to form new tumors in other organs. The spread of cancer is called metastasis.

Either way, whether a cancer is localized or spreading, it can be defined by its staging.

Over the years, the common elements of staging systems for cancer have evolved. They continue to change even today as scientists learn more about cancer. Some staging systems cover many types of cancer; others are specific to a particular type.

The common elements considered in most staging systems include:

- Location of the primary tumor
- Tumor size and number of tumors
- Lymph node involvement (spread of cancer into lymph nodes)
- Cell type and tumor grade (how closely the cancer cells resemble normal tissue)
- Presence or absence of metastasis

TNM: The Cancer Reporter

The TNM system is one of the most commonly used staging systems. Most medical facilities use it as their main method for cancer reporting. It is based on the extent of the tumor (T), the extent of the spreading to the lymph nodes (N), and the presence of metastasis (M). A number is added to each letter to indicate the size or extent of the tumor and the extent of spread.

Tumors (T) and lymph nodes (L) designated as X means that the tumor or lymph nodes can't be evaluated. Tumors (T) and lymph nodes (L) designated as 0 show no evidence of tumor or lymph nodes.

The numbers 1, 2, 3, and 4 indicate the size and extent of the primary tumor or the number/extent of the tumor's spread into regional lymph nodes.

Metastasis (M) designated as MX cannot be evaluated. A designation of M0 means that the cancer has not spread to other parts of the body. M1 means that the cancer has spread to distant parts of the body.

For example, breast cancer T3 N2 M0 refers to a large tumor (T3) that has spread outside the breast to nearby lymph nodes (N2) but not to other parts of the body (M0). Prostate cancer T2 N0 M0 means that the tumor (T2) is located only in the prostate and has not spread to the lymph nodes (N0) or any other part of the body (M0).

For many cancers, TNM combinations correspond to one of five stages. Criteria for stages differ for different types of cancer. For example, bladder cancer T3 N0 M0 is stage III; however, colon cancer T3 N0 M0 is stage II.

Rasheen Davis, author of *The Chemo Room: My Journey Through Fear, Hope and Survival,* found out that staging is one of the most important numbers in a patient's life. It helps the doctor make a prognosis and plan appropriate treatment. Staging helps healthcare providers and researchers exchange information about patients. It also provides a common terminology to evaluate treatment results.

"Like a golfer," Rasheen says, "you want your score to be low, like I. Never IV."

How Do I Explain It?

A diagnosis of cancer is a lot for anyone to digest, to say the least. When taking in and trying to process an onslaught of new information—let alone all the emotions that come with it—any previous experience with being sick, or taking care of someone who is, makes little to no difference.

And when you must explain your condition to others in your life—family, friends, colleagues, and neighbors—the task can be daunting. That's why having the right information is so essential—to help you understand what you're going through and to make it easier to communicate all of it with the important people in your life.

So whether it's breast cancer or any of the other cancers that are gender specific to a woman, we encourage you to be patient and keep reading because you will find much of what you will need to know—and ask your medical team about—as you proceed through this journey.

KEY POINTS TO REMEMBER

✓ Reimagining cancer is made possible by research advances.

✓ Precision diagnoses and targeted treatments allow us to treat many cancers more effectively and with fewer side effects than in the past.

✓ Ask your doctor seventeen crucial questions.

✓ Grading and staging of cancer is an essential part of the diagnostic process and provide information on your prognosis and guide your treatment.

✓ Your attitude plays a big part in how you deal with this entire process.

I Am a Cancer Patient

I am a cancer patient,
a mother, a wife, a daughter, and a friend.
I have a career and goals and a past filled with memories.
Sometimes, I wonder who will care for my children if I am gone,
Sometimes, I am certain I will live forever.

I am a cancer patient,
a survivor, an inspiration, and an advocate.
I have endured medical procedures and treatments
and felt exposed to total strangers in whose hands I lay my future.
I have moments of complete confusion and moments of total
  understanding,
nights of restless sleep and days of doubt and rage.

I am a cancer patient,
skilled at disguising any signs of illness with wigs and hats and makeup
  and smiles,
but do not be fooled—I am afraid.

I am a cancer patient.
viewed with pity and awe and a certain misunderstanding
by those who have not shared my journey.
I enjoy peaceful moments amidst the uncertainty
because I am acutely aware of life's preciousness.

I am a cancer patient,
a product of challenge.
I am thankful for the side effects that have helped me become
a better mother, a wife, a daughter, and a friend.
I am blessed to live life large.

—Amy Breitmann

2 FINDING HOPE IN A SHADOW OF FEAR: What You Need to Know About Breast Cancer

Obviously, it wasn't meant for me to die of cancer at forty.
Every day my life surprises me, just like
my cancer diagnosis surprised me.
But you roll with it. That's our job as humans.

—Edie Falco, as told to *health.com*

Discrimination? No. Education? Yes.

Jamie Farris was only twenty-five years old and a single mother of two little boys when she was diagnosed with breast cancer. She tried to convince her doctor that she couldn't work it into her schedule, that he could simply not tell her that she had it. "I'm in my twenties, for God's sake," she shouted. "No one my age gets cancer. What am I going to tell my boys?"

Seven weeks later, after what was thought to be successful surgery and several awful rounds of chemotherapy, Jamie came home one day and headed straight for the bathroom to throw up. She was ready to give in, to end it right there, until one of her sons found her crying and brought her back to her senses. Jamie realized then that she had so much to live for, and after flushing a handful of pills down the toilet, she put her life back together.

Jamie's story is not unusual. Cancer does not discriminate. It can happen to anyone at any time and does not care about age, color, religion, or income. The best thing we can do when it does occur, and which helped Jamie immeasurably, is to educate ourselves about our bodies and what happens to them when cancer appears, apparently out of the blue, for no good reason.

Basic Anatomy and Function

Breasts consist mostly of organized collections of fat cells, medically known as adipose tissue, which are arranged into twelve to twenty sections called lobes, which are made up of smaller units called lobules—the glands that produce milk. Thin tubes called ducts carry the milk from the lobules to the nipple.

In addition to fat cells, the breast also contains a network of ligaments and fibrous connective tissue that help support it, as well as nerves to provide sensation; blood and lymphatic vessels to bring oxygen and nutrients; and infection-fighting cells, lymph nodes, and lymphatic channels that drain and filter body fluids and cells. Glandular tissue of the breast is not uniformly distributed, and there tends to be more in the upper outer portion of the breast. This is why many women complain of pain in this area just before their periods.

This is also the site of approximately half of all breast cancers.

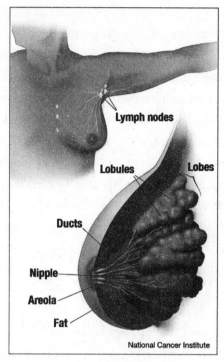

Breast Anatomy

Causes of Breast Cancer

In the United States, breast cancer is the second most common cancer in women after skin cancer. Each year, about 230,000 cases of breast cancer are diagnosed in women and about 2,300 in men.

Cancer is caused by mutations in the DNA that makes up our genes. Human beings have about 20,000 genes; but only about 160 of these are directly involved in cancer, and only a handful are considered to be the main "drivers" of breast cancer.

DNA mutations can occur in either *germ* or *somatic* cells of the body. Germ cells are either sperm or eggs, and are responsible for transmitting genes from parent to child. Somatic cells refer to all of the other cells in your body. Mutations in somatic cells of the breast are the cause of the vast majority (90 to 95 percent) of breast cancers. These cancers do not run in families; in other words, they are not the result of a predisposing, hereditary condition.

Hereditary cancers, on the other hand, are defined by mutations in germ cells, and the risk of developing cancer is passed between generations. Hereditary cancers are often part of familial syndromes that transmit the risk of developing several types of cancer, for example, cancers of the breast and ovary. We explore hereditary breast cancer in much greater detail in Chapter 3.

Diagnosing Breast Cancer: Your Personal Responsibility

The diagnosis and treatment of breast cancer almost always "takes a village" and may involve as many as five to eight different types of doctors and other specialized medical professionals. These include primary care physicians and gynecologists, radiologists, surgeons, pathologists, medical oncologists, and radiation oncologists. Specialized oncology nurses are critical members of the healthcare team, as are genetic counselors. We will describe the roles and responsibilities of these different specialists as we progress through patients' cancer journeys in this chapter and in Chapters 3 and 4.

However, the most important person in the diagnosis of breast cancer is the woman herself. Monthly breast self-exams are vital, and being aware of when to have screening mammograms (see below) are powerful tools that every woman should use to take charge of her health. Personal responsibility also means learning about ways to prevent cancer: acquiring knowledge about environmental and genetic risk factors for developing the disease.

MY JOURNEY

As soon as I was diagnosed, a friend of mine—a breast cancer *survivor*—said that making myself the priority would be the most important thing I could do to ensure a successful recovery.

As a nurse and mother, I'm quite familiar with taking care of others, but it was soon clear that I wasn't terribly adept at doing the same thing for myself. I had to admit that I was lucky I even got diagnosed as early as I did. I knew this way of living was not okay, that my world had been turned upside down, and if I didn't start looking out for number one, I would end up useless to anyone else.

Right then and there, as soon as my friend helped me see the light, I decided to start giving myself permission to take care of me first, which meant paying less attention to the world around me and all of the daily distractions and demands. That was my first step toward healing.

Robin (Santa Fe, New Mexico)

Signs and Symptoms

- A lump or thickening in or near the breast or in the underarm area
- A change in the size or shape of the breast
- A dimple or puckering in the skin of the breast
- A nipple turned inward into the breast
- Fluid, other than breast milk, from the nipple, especially if it's bloody
- Scaly, red, or swollen skin on the breast, nipple, or areola (dark area around the nipple)
- Dimples in the breast resembling the skin of an orange, called *peau d'orange*

If any of these signs or symptoms occurs, a woman should schedule the first available appointment with her primary care physician or gynecologist, who will perform a physical examination and interpret the findings in terms of a clinical diagnosis.

> **NOTE to PATIENT:**
> Make sure to let your doctor know
> if cancer of any type seems to run in your family.

The clinical diagnosis may determine that the patient is either likely or unlikely to have cancer and may need further tests, which usually consist of the following:

- *Diagnostic mammography* (see The Mammogram Controversy in this chapter) or ultrasound imaging (see Joan Lunden, also in this chapter).
- *Surgical biopsy*, also known as a fine-needle aspiration, which is used to obtain tissue and cells for pathologic diagnosis

Melissa Etheridge and the Importance of Self-Exams

Rock singer Melissa Etheridge first came to prominence in 1993 when she won her first Grammy for her single "Ain't It Heavy." Later that year, she released her mainstream breakthrough album, *Yes I Am.* The album contained three top-forty hits, including "I'm Not the Only One" and "Come to My Window," for which she won a second Grammy.

In 2004 Etheridge was riding high with her successful career. Etheridge released *Lucky,* her eighth album. She was in a new relationship with Tammy Lynn Michaels and had received another Grammy nomination. In October she was near the end of her summer concert tour when she felt a lump in her left breast while showering.

"I was like, 'Whoa!' And it was large!" she told *AARP* magazine at the time. "That little voice in the back of my head started going, 'Is it cancer? Your father died of cancer. Your aunt died of cancer. Your grandmother, too. Your mother had cancer. Your cousin. Cancer. Cancer.' You just can't quiet the voice."

She tried telling herself it was just a cyst. But the lump was not a cyst. It was breast cancer, and she underwent a lumpectomy to remove the four-centimeter (1.5 inch) tumor. The cancer had also spread to something called a sentinel lymph node. Since the lymphatic system drains fluid and cells from parts of our bodies, including the breast, a lymph node that is closest to a tumor acts as a soldier or guard that stands and keeps watch. In this case, that soldier reported that the cancer had begun to spread. Ms. Etheridge was therefore treated with chemotherapy followed by radiation therapy.

Melissa made a return to the stage at the 2005 Grammy Awards. Still bald from chemotherapy, she belted out Janis Joplin's "Piece of My Heart." The moving performance became a symbol of empowerment for women struggling with and surviving breast cancer.

Etheridge has remained cancer-free for ten years, which she attributes to major changes in her life, including what she eats and how she deals with stress and making critical choices.

Mammograms: Why the Controversy?

In 2009 Melissa Etheridge was one of the many celebrities who spoke out about new proposed guidelines for using mammography as a screening test for breast cancer. These guidelines caused quite a controversy because the medical science had become confused and comingled with political debates about healthcare reform. This caused massive confusion and the whole issue became sensationalized.

We'll describe the medical science and the controversy in more detail later, but first let's answer an essential question: What exactly is a mammogram?

A mammogram is an X-ray image of the breast. It can be used as a tool to screen for breast cancer in women who have no signs or symptoms of the disease. Screening mammograms usually involve two X-ray images of each breast. These make it possible to detect tumors that are not large enough to be felt by the woman or her doctor. Screening mammograms can also find micro-calcifications (tiny deposits of calcium) that sometimes indicate the presence of cancer.

Mammograms can also be used to check for breast cancer after a lump or other sign or symptom of the disease has been found. This type of mammogram is called a diagnostic mammogram, which can also be used to evaluate changes found during a screening mammogram, or to view breast tissue when it is difficult to obtain a screening mammogram because of special circumstances, such as the presence of breast implants.

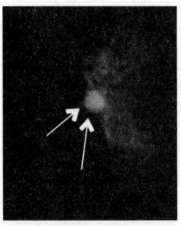

Breast Cancer Found on Mammogram
Source: *CelebrityDiagnosis.com*

A diagnostic mammogram is different from a screening mammogram in that additional X-ray images are needed in a diagnostic mammogram to see the breast from several angles. The technician can also magnify a suspicious area to obtain a more detailed picture. This can help the doctor make an accurate diagnosis.

The major benefit of screening mammography is that early detection of breast cancer means that treatment can be started earlier in the course of the disease, possibly before it has spread. Once again, early detection can make a huge difference in subsequent treatment.

So what was all the fuss about back in 2009?

In March of that year, two statistical researchers, Charlotte Ahern and Yu Shen, published an important article about their studies of the cost-effectiveness of mammography and breast exams and how they compared with existing guidelines. At the time, three major cancer organizations in the United States had different guidelines, and as a result there was no consensus about which guidelines were to be considered best.

The American Cancer Society (ACS) recommended an annual mammography for women forty years and older and a breast exam every three years beginning at age twenty and switching to every year at age forty. The National Cancer Institute (NCI) recommended a mammography every one to two years. The U.S. Preventive Services Task Force (USPSTF) recommended a mammography every two years for women fifty to seventy-four years old and considered it an "individualized" decision to screen between ages forty and forty-nine.

Confusing? For many women and doctors it was—and continues to be.

Doctors Ahern and Shen set out to gather evidence about the cost-effectiveness of these three strategies, compared with other combinations of mammograms and breast exams. As a result of their research and analysis, they suggested a more cost-effective strategy would be to recommend mammograms every other year, alternating with breast exams in the non-mammogram years.

This simple suggestion, backed up by careful statistical analysis, proved to be a match that lit a firestorm of controversy. It was just a coincidence, but publication of this study in March 2009 coincided with a health summit convened by President Obama to study issues relating to the Affordable Care Act (ACA) legislation—also known as Obamacare—to be presented to Congress later that year.

Both advocates and opponents of the ACA seized on Ahern and Shen's study to support their own positions. This led to a tremendous amount of misinformation about the study that was disseminated to the public. As they often do, good-intentioned but perhaps not well-informed celebrities became vocal about the subject.

For example, songwriter and actress Olivia Newton-John said, "We are being put back in the Dark Ages again. We are not data; we are human beings."

Actress and businesswoman Jaclyn Smith was shocked, declaring, "They want to abandon proven therapies. It's wrong."

Because Ms. Newton-John and Ms. Smith were both breast-cancer survivors, their statements had a huge impact on public perceptions of both the medical and political issues.

Two other breast cancer survivors and friends since 1988, Melissa Etheridge and Sheryl Crow had more thoughtful and helpful reactions: "We women have to start looking at ourselves and taking back control of our health," Ms. Etheridge said. "It's understanding your health, so when someone tells you that you don't need a mammogram until you're fifty, you know that, and you take charge of that decision."

Ms. Crow said, "I encourage all women everywhere to advocate for themselves and for their future. See your doctor and be proactive about your health."

Mammograms: When and How Often?

As of 2015, the American Cancer Society and the United States Preventative Services Task Force had not changed their breast cancer screening guidelines since 2009. The National Cancer Institute now highlights the importance of both mammography and breast exams and also points out mammography's risks.

It's important to realize that these recommendations are based on statistics that apply to "average" women. But not every woman has average risks, and only you and your primary care doctor, informed by your current health and family medical history, can determine what choices are right for you.

The National Cancer Institute provides a Breast Cancer Risk Calculator on their website[2] that may help you decide how to manage your health. We also discuss the specific risks of screening mammograms in Chapter 13.

——————————— MY JOURNEY ———————————

As a radiologist specializing in breast imaging, I know cancer when I see it. I was forty-one when I viewed my own mammogram and knew immediately what I was looking at. Lucky for me, I had started screening mammograms a year earlier when I was forty because otherwise, after surgery, chemo, and radiation, I may not be alive today to share my story with my patients. Hopefully when I do, I am able to ease their anxiety and reassure them that a good outcome is quite possible.

Lea (Miami, Florida)

---

2. *www.cancer.gov/bcrisktool/*

"Lucky" Accidents:
Giuliana Rancic and Wanda Sykes

When patients in the midst of being tested or treated for other conditions are found to have cancer, doctors sometimes call this an "incidental finding." When this occurs, it can be considered lucky in the sense that the cancer might have otherwise gone undetected until it reached a more advanced and dangerous state.

Back in 2011, when *E! News* host Giuliana Rancic and her husband, Bill Rancic, winner of *The Apprentice*, were struggling with infertility, they shared the experience on their reality show, *Giuliana and Bill*. In October of that year, the couple was seen heading to Denver for a third try at in vitro fertilization (IVF). As part of the pre-IVF workup, the infertility doctor insisted that Giuliana have a mammogram because the hormones used to treat infertility can also make any existing cancers worse.

Rancic's doctors detected an early-stage cancer, so Rancic underwent bilateral lumpectomies. Unfortunately, the pathologist's report revealed that the surgery had not removed all of the cancer in one breast, leaving her with two options: undergo another lumpectomy followed by radiation therapy and anti-estrogen therapy or accept bilateral mastectomies.

Rancic opted for the latter, a much more extensive procedure but one that would lower her risk of subsequent breast cancers. Another consideration, which may have influenced her decision, was that if she had chosen to have the lumpectomy, the antiestrogen therapy would delay for several years any possibility of having a child.

The surgery was successful, and, in August 2012, the couple welcomed their son, Duke, born via a gestational carrier.

A little earlier, in 2011, comedienne Wanda Sykes underwent surgery to reduce the size of her breasts because, according to her, they "got in my way" and gave her back pain. However, when pathologists examined a sampling of breast tissue, they found that she had ductal carcinoma *in situ* (DCIS) in the left breast.

Despite that all of the cancer had been removed during the breast reduction surgery, Sykes made the dramatic decision to have both breasts removed. She points out that she has a strong family history of breast cancer. She was also afraid she would be unable to keep up with the frequent monitoring (mammogram and breast MRI every three months) she would have to maintain to make sure the cancer hadn't returned.

Meet Your Pathologist—or Not

The medical process of a pathology diagnosis is the gold standard by which cancer is diagnosed and upon which treatment plans are based. The specialist who performs this diagnosis is called a pathologist. Unfortunately, he or she is often the only member of a care team—and the most important doctor—the patient will probably *never* meet.

Pathologists are medical doctors who spend an additional four to five years after medical school learning the field of laboratory medicine. Their work includes detecting and analyzing tissue biopsies, blood samples, urine samples, and other types of specimens collected from patients. They issue written reports directly to the pathology department or clinical laboratory that is responsible for testing the samples and reporting back to other members of the care team.

It's the job of the pathologist to diagnose whether the biopsy specimen represents cancer or something else, such as an infection or fibrocystic disease. If the pathologist determines that the specimen is cancer, he or she will then report precisely what type of cancer it is, a finding that carries critical implications for subsequent treatment.

Although many pathologists don't routinely interact directly with patients, this doesn't mean that the patient can't ask to meet or talk with the pathologist whose expertise is one of the most critical factors in a cancer patient's prognosis and care.

One extremely important step in the process that can affect the accuracy of the pathologic diagnosis is how the patient's tissue specimen is handled and processed during the time between its surgical removal and its arrival in the pathology lab. The details of tissue processing and transport are called pre-analytic variables. If certain strict protocols are not followed, this process can result in a missed or incorrect diagnosis.

We recommend that, if and when you become a patient and are asked to sign a consent form for a biopsy or other type of surgery, you inquire about which pathologist will be responsible for handling your specimen and whether there are any special protocols for processing your tissue based on the type of cancer you are suspected of having.

In case of unexpected findings at the time of surgery, your pathologist may be called to the operating room to consult with your surgeon in determining how the specimen should be handled. Therefore, it is essential that you speak up about these matters. Once again, this is a situation where assuming personal responsibility is in your best interest.

This is also because pathology, like many other sciences, does not always yield perfectly accurate results. While the practice of pathology relies on science, it also involves human judgment and experience, meaning mistakes can be made that may result in an incorrect or misleading diagnosis.

Last year, Johns Hopkins Hospital in Baltimore reviewed tissue samples from 6,000 cancer patients nationwide and found one out of every seventy-one cases was misdiagnosed. In one case, emblematic of many they discovered, a biopsy was labeled cancerous when in fact it was found not to be. They also found incorrect classifications in up to one out of five cases.

This type of error in judgment—in how fast or how far the cancer had spread—can significantly affect a patient's prognosis and care.

Dr. Jonathan Epstein of Johns Hopkins Hospital concurs: "That can change whether a patient gets no treatment versus surgery versus radiation, and if they get surgery or radiation, which type."

According to this study and others, errors can be made in any biopsy, but they are found most often in tissue samples from the skin, prostate, breast, and female reproductive tract.

According to Dr. Leonard Zwelling of the MD Anderson Cancer Center in Houston, "We really still make the diagnosis pretty much the way we did for the last fifty years. It has to come down to looking at a piece of the tumor on a slide by a pathologist."

NOTE to PATIENT:
Get a second opinion from an expert pathologist.

Your pathologist's report is part of your medical record, and it is your right to obtain a copy of this report. Sometimes you may also want to obtain a second opinion from another pathologist with special expertise in your type of cancer (see the Rita Wilson story in this chapter).

Multiple Types of Breast Cancer: Why Does It Matter?

Ductal carcinoma *in situ* (DCIS) is the most common type of noninvasive breast cancer. Some experts consider DCIS to be a premalignant condition. *Ductal* means that the cancer starts inside cells that line the milk ducts. *In situ* is Latin for "in its original place," and means the cancer has not spread through or beyond the duct.

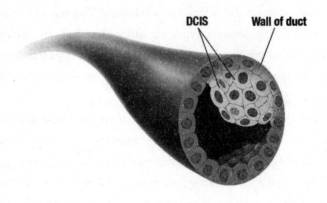

DCIS
Source: The National Cancer Institute

Simply put, DCIS is a group of abnormal cancer cells in a milk duct that remains limited to the duct. In 20 to 30 percent of cases, DCIS may become invasive cancer and spread to other tissues, although it is not known yet how to predict which lesions will become invasive.

Breast cancer can also begin in the cells of the lobules and in other tissues in the breast.

Invasive breast cancer is a type that has spread from where it began in the ducts or lobules into the surrounding tissue. This is when cancer has spread beyond its original place and is no longer referred to as DCIS.

Some controversy exists about whether DCIS should be considered cancer at all and if it should be treated in all women. We explore more of this later in this chapter in a story about celebrity chef Sandra Lee.

Defining specific cancers is traditionally done using two main features or characteristics: the anatomic location where the cancer occurs, for example breast, ovary, cervix, and what the malignant tissue looks like under a microscope, a view referred to as microscopic anatomy, morphology/histopathology.

Based on the latter criteria, there are about thirty-five types of breast cancer, according to the *WHO Classification of Tumours of the Breast*, Volume 4.[3] Many of these types are quite rare. But, in any event, these traditional classifications, based on a cancer's appearance under the microscope, have increasingly less bearing on modern treatment choices.

Since the late 1990s (as described in Chapter 1), these diseases we call cancer have been undergoing a fundamental rethinking based on molecular features too small to be seen using a normal microscope. Most often, these features are abnormal versions of genes (DNA) or proteins that are the actual cause(s) of cancer or that drive a tumor's dangerously uncontrolled growth and behavior.

Practically speaking, from a drug treatment point of view, there are three major types of breast cancer. They differ in terms of the best drugs to treat them, so it's critically important for a pathologist to be as precise as possible in his or her diagnosis.

ER/PR-Positive (ER/PR+) Breast Cancer

This is the most common category of breast cancer affecting about 65 percent of women with the disease. ER stands for estrogen receptor, PR stands for progesterone receptor.

HER2-Positive (HER2+) Breast Cancer

About 20 percent of women with breast cancers are in this category. HER2 stands for human epidermal growth factor receptor number 2. The HER2 gene is amplified in this form of breast cancer and acts like an accelerator for cancer cells.

---

3. *http://apps.who.int/bookorders/anglais/detart1.jsp?codlan=1&codcol=70&codcch=4004.*

Triple-Negative Breast Cancer (TNBC)

This type of cancer lacks the three biomarkers (ER/PR and HER2) that define the other two types. About 15 percent of breast cancers are of the TNBC type, which occur more frequently in younger and premenopausal women and is highly prevalent in African American and Hispanic women. This cancer type is similar to tumors that are caused by mutations in the BRCA1 gene (Chapter 3).

Unlike for ER/PR+ and HER2+ cancers, currently no FDA approved, targeted drugs are available for TNBC. However, new immunotherapies, described later in this chapter, are being tested and may be a treatment option in the not too distant future.

TNBC can be more aggressive and difficult to treat. TNBC is more likely to spread and recur. It has also been found to be more responsive to traditional chemotherapy than many other forms of cancer.

Detecting these types using special tests in a medical laboratory is a process called companion diagnostics. Companion refers to the fact that precision medicine drugs—aka targeted therapies—to treat each type go hand in hand with the presence or absence of their companion biomarkers, which are often cellular proteins, called receptors.

Ultrasound Imaging

Since consistency of breast tissue varies from woman to woman, and even between two breasts of the same individual, this technology is especially vital for the information it provides, and it is easy to administer because of its noninvasive nature.

The glandular portion of breast tissue has a firm, somewhat nubby feel to it, while the surrounding fat is typically soft. It is exactly this difference in the feel and density of these two tissues that allow a mammogram to differentiate them.

The breast tissue of younger women tends to be denser, with more glandular tissue and less fat. Over time, especially after the loss of estrogen that comes with menopause, the glandular tissue shrivels (involutes) and is replaced by fatty tissue.

Dense breasts make it more difficult to detect breast cancer on a mammogram. This is because dense breast tissue can look white/gray on a mammogram—the same as cancer, which is indicated in the following diagram.

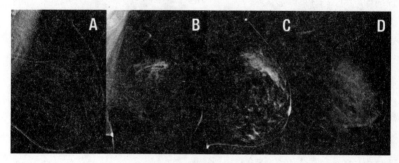

Variation in Breast Density
Source: Courtesy of Dr. Wendie Berg, *densebreast-info.org/*

Some physicians use ultrasound to supplement a routine mammography in women with dense breasts. Ultrasound, or sonography, uses sound waves to look inside a part of the body. An instrument called a transducer is rubbed across the skin, which is lubricated with a special ultrasound gel. No radiation is involved, which is why it is safe to use in pregnant women.

Breast ultrasound is often used to evaluate breast problems that are found during a screening or diagnostic mammogram, or during a physical exam. Ultrasound can help distinguish between a cyst (fluid-filled sac) and a solid mass.

Research has shown that ultrasound is not a good tool for mass screening for breast cancer, as there is an unacceptable rate of false negatives and positives. According to the American Cancer Society, clinical trials are currently examining the potential benefits and risks of using breast ultrasound along with screening mammograms in women with dense breasts and a higher risk of breast cancer.

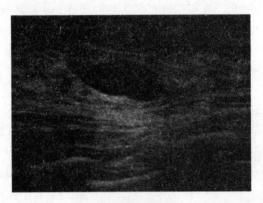

Simple Breast Cyst
Source: © Nevit Dilmen

Joan Lunden: The Benefits of Ultrasound

In June 2014, former *Good Morning America* cohost Joan Lunden revealed that she had been diagnosed with breast cancer. Lunden had a normal screening mammogram, but because of her history of dense breast tissue, she was also screened with a breast ultrasound, which ultimately revealed the tumor. A biopsy and pathologic diagnosis determined that she was suffering from triple-negative breast cancer.

After nine months of treatment, including sixteen rounds of chemotherapy, a lumpectomy, and six weeks of radiation, in June 2015 Lunden's doctors declared her cancer-free.

Throughout the process she stayed in the public eye, hoping to use her cancer journey as an opportunity to inspire others to protect their health.

She kept a video diary of her treatment, did a series of reports on the *Today* show, and even appeared bald on the cover of *People* magazine.

Lunden has a streaming network dedicated to breast cancer and women's health and wellness issues called *Alive with Joan Lunden*.

When asked by the *Today* show what she learned from her experience, Lunden responded, "I went from being a patient to being a survivor to being an advocate and really now a bit of an educator. When you get hit with something like this and you become part of this breast cancer world, it's like a sorority that you don't really want to join, and the initiation process is not so great. But, boy, once you're in it, it's so powerful and so compassionate. Everybody just comes to your support and aid, and the response I got on social media was so overwhelming and so healing that I really was taught the lesson of how important the power of support is to a patient."

> **NOTE to PATIENT:**
> Ultrasound should not replace the mammogram
> for breast cancer screening.
> It may be used as an additional test to tell whether
> a mass seen on a mammogram
> or felt by a physician is a cyst or solid mass,
> or as a supplemental test for women
> with particularly dense breasts.

MY JOURNEY

I have been doing my own breast checking for years. When I turned forty, I found a lump in my right breast and immediately scheduled a mammogram, which confirmed a strong probability of cancer. A biopsy confirmed it. To make a long story short, I had a lumpectomy, nodes removed, and more rounds of chemo and radiation than I can remember. My advice to women is to start checking your breasts as soon as they begin to appear! Get into the practice! My doctor told me I was lucky to discover my lump before it spread. I wish the same for all women who are dealing with the same possibilities!

Tamara (Bloomington, Indiana)

Sandra Lee: Cancer-Free and Ready to Go

Popular TV chef (*Semi-Homemade Cooking*) and author Sandra Lee, forty-nine, was diagnosed with ductal carcinoma *in situ* (DCIS) in March 2015. A routine annual mammogram detected this early-stage cancer. Lee originally had a lumpectomy, but the surgical edges were not totally free of cancer, so doctors advised her that she would also need six to eight weeks of daily radiation therapy. Her physicians also recommended that she consider having a mastectomy.

As Lee told *Good Morning America* co-anchor Robin Roberts, "I said, 'Okay. If I'm going to have a mastectomy, am I supposed to just get one done?' Both the radiologist and the doctor said, 'You're a ticking time bomb.' And they both said, 'You need to get them both done.'"

Lee underwent a bilateral mastectomy in May, with a lot of support from her longtime partner, New York Governor Andrew Cuomo, who took a break from his demanding schedule to be with Sandra after her surgery.

In September 2015, four months after her diagnosis, Lee once again went to *Good Morning America* to talk to Robin Roberts, this time with good news.

"The beautiful thing about early-stage cancer," she said, "is it gives you every option in the world, and that is what I took. My doctors have said that I am cancer-free and ready to go."

Treating DCIS

According to the American Cancer Society, about 60,000 cases of DCIS are diagnosed in the United States each year, accounting for about one out of every five new breast cancer cases. Less than 10 percent of DCIS are detected by breast exam while 80 percent are diagnosed by mammography.

According to National Comprehensive Cancer Network (NCCN) guidelines, treatment options for DCIS include mastectomy, lumpectomy with radiation therapy (XRT), and lumpectomy alone with possible hormonal treatment for ER/PR+ cancers.

This next chart shows how often these various treatment approaches were used in 2015.

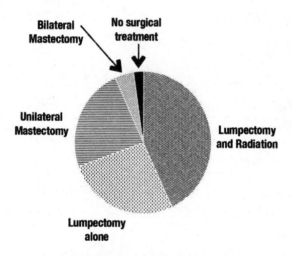

Frequency of Treatment Options for DCIS
Source: *CelebrityDiagnosis.com*

NOTE to PATIENT:
Fewer than 1 in 10 women treated for DCIS
will die as a result of their disease.

Can Cancer Be Eliminated Just by
Changing Its Name?

In the summer of 2013, about 32,000 American women carried the diagnosis of breast cancer. When they woke up on the morning of August 28, the cancer was gone. Was this some kind of miracle? Not really. On that hot summer day, a group of medical experts published their views in the *Journal of American Medical Association* (*JAMA*) that the disease these women had (DCIS) should no longer be called cancer at all. In other words, they eliminated a frightening diagnosis by simply changing its name.[4]

How could they do that?

In 70 to 80 percent of cases, DCIS will not progress to invasive disease. The authors of the *JAMA* article, including breast cancer surgeon Dr. Laura Esserman, said, "The term 'cancer' often invokes the specter of an inexorably lethal condition," and that the term *cancer* should be reserved for conditions with a "reasonable likelihood of lethal progression if left untreated."

The *JAMA* authors pointed out that DCIS and some other conditions currently known as cancer are precancerous conditions, identified by potential over-screening and thereby subject to potential overtreatment. They recommended a number of actions to reimagine some types of cancer as less dangerous and less frightening types of disease.

As Dr. Otis Brawly put it, "We need a twenty-first-century definition of cancer instead of a nineteenth-century definition, which is what we've been using."

Dr. Brawley is the Chief Medical Officer of the American Cancer Society and was not associated with the *JAMA* article, but he did tell

---

4. *https://www.ncbi.nlm.nih.gov/pubmed/19843904; http://jama.jamanetwork.com/article.aspx? articleid=184747*

National Public Radio's *Tell Me More,* "What we're trying to do is spare some people the harms associated with unnecessary treatment. And there are a lot of people who are demanding unnecessary treatment. There are also a lot of doctors who don't understand that not every cancer is highly aggressive and there's a wide spectrum of cancers. We are helping those doctors understand, helping the patients understand."

Rita Wilson: The Importance of Getting a Second Opinion

In April 2015, actress Rita Wilson announced that she had recently undergone a bilateral mastectomy with reconstructive surgery to treat breast cancer.

"I have taken a leave from the play *Fish in the Dark* to deal with a personal health issue," she told *People* magazine. "Last week, with my husband [two-time Academy Award–winner Tom Hanks] by my side, and with the love and support of family and friends, I underwent a bilateral mastectomy and reconstruction for breast cancer after a diagnosis of invasive lobular carcinoma. I am recovering and, most importantly, expected to make a full recovery. Why? Because I caught this early, have excellent doctors, and because I got a second opinion."

Wilson went on to explain that doctors have been following her for "an underlying condition of LCIS (lobular carcinoma *in situ*), which has been vigilantly monitored through yearly mammograms and breast MRIs. Recently, after two surgical breast biopsies, PCIS (pleomorphic carcinoma *in situ*) was discovered."

The adjective *pleomorphic* refers to the fact that the sizes and shapes of breast cells are highly variable when viewed through a microscope. *In situ* is a Latin phrase that translates literally to "on site" or "in position."

In all her interviews, Wilson stressed the importance of getting a second opinion.

"My gut told me that was the thing to do. A different pathologist found invasive lobular carcinoma. His diagnosis of cancer was confirmed by yet another pathologist. I share this to educate others that a second opinion is critical to your health. You have nothing to lose if both opinions match up for the good, and everything to gain if something that was missed is found, which does happen. Early diagnosis is key."

> **NOTE to PATIENT:**
> Early diagnosis is key!

The surgery didn't keep Wilson sidelined for long. She returned to Broadway in May. Her stepson (and actor) Colin Hanks told *Entertainment Tonight* that Wilson is now cancer-free. Wilson gives her husband a lot of credit in aiding her recovery. She told the *New York Times*, "You never know how your spouse is going to react in a situation like this. I was so amazed, so blown away by the care my husband gave me. It was such a normal, intimate time."

What's a Guy to Do?

Marc Silver, author of *Breast Cancer Husband: How to Help Your Wife (and Yourself) During Diagnosis, Treatment and Beyond*, had his hands full in 2001 when his wife was diagnosed with bilateral breast cancer—a lump in each breast. He tried to be the best caregiver he knew how to be, but it certainly wasn't easy. "Being a typical guy, I screwed up," Marc wrote in an essay that appeared in Chicken Soup for the Soul's *The Cancer Book: 101 Stories of Courage, Support and Love.*

"I played the denial game. I rooted for her relentlessly. Eventually, I got the hang of how to help (in a nutshell: don't try to fix things, just shut up and listen)."

Marc is not alone. Many men, when their partners are diagnosed with breast cancer (or any type, for that matter), find themselves balancing multiple challenges at the same time, from insurance company roadblocks to endless appointments to a terrible new fear of the unknown.

"Marsha had to face her own mortality," Marc said, "which is a heck of a lot more daunting than what I had to face: the unspoken 'what if' that hovers when a loved one has cancer. Unlike me, Marsha never really could escape all of these worries because her body always reminded her of what she was going through. I could sympathize with her traumas. But I couldn't even begin to imagine the courage it takes to submit to the seemingly endless (and endlessly painful) treatments. I'm not sure I would have been as brave as Marsha. During her chemo months, I had a dream in which I had to have a chemotherapy infusion. I was a total chicken. I wouldn't let them stick that needle in my veins. I awoke in a cold sweat. But it was just a dream."

From Marc and all the spouses of those coping with breast cancer, we might learn a central lesson: it's plenty hard on both parties, and the most important thing is to keep an open heart and mind.

Explaining LCIS (Lobular Carcinoma *in Situ*)

Lobular carcinoma *in situ* (LCIS) is diagnosed when abnormal cells grow inside the lobules of the breast but have not spread to nearby tissue or beyond. LCIS is not considered invasive breast cancer, as it tends to remain in place (*in situ*). However, those diagnosed with LCIS are at a higher risk of developing breast cancer. Women with LCIS are considered eight to ten times more likely to develop invasive cancer, which can occur as either invasive lobular or ductal carcinoma.

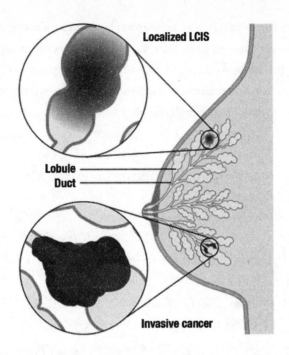

Lobular Carcinoma in Situ and Invasive Lobular Carcinoma
Source: Cancer Research UK *commons.wikimedia.org/w/index.php?curid=34333551*

Special breast cancer screening guidelines exist for women with LCIS. They should have breast exams every six to twelve months and get a yearly mammogram. Several groups, such as the American Cancer Society and the National Comprehensive Cancer Network, also recommend that women with LCIS (or those with a personal history of breast cancer, ductal carcinoma *in situ* [DCIS], atypical ductal hyperplasia [ADH], or atypical lobular hyperplasia [ALH]) speak with their doctors about having an MRI scan as well.

Some women diagnosed with LCIS are treated with the antiestrogen drugs tamoxifen or raloxifene to try to lower their risk of breast cancer. Tamoxifen has been shown to be slightly more effective in cancer prevention than raloxifene, but it comes with the risk of greater side effects. A substantial amount of information is online pertaining to tamoxifen, and we recommend you do your due diligence before signing on for this treatment. Once again, the question you can be asking goes like this: Is it right for me?

Invasive Lobular Breast Cancer (ILC)

This is the second most common type of breast cancer. Approximately 10 percent of women with breast cancer have lobular carcinoma, which begins in a breast lobule, while the rest have invasive ductal carcinoma, which begins in the milk ducts.

Choosing a treatment plan for ILC depends on the same factors as other breast cancers:

- The stage of the cancer (the size of the tumor and whether it is in the breast only or has spread to lymph nodes or other places in the body)
- Estrogen receptor and progesterone receptor levels in the tumor tissue
- Human epidermal growth factor type 2 receptor (HER2/neu) levels in the tumor tissue
- If the tumor tissue is triple-negative (cells that do not have estrogen receptors, progesterone receptors, or abnormal levels of HER2/neu)
- The speed of tumor growth
- The likelihood of recurrence
- A woman's age and general health
- If a woman is still having menstrual periods
- Whether the cancer is newly diagnosed or has recurred

MY JOURNEY

I will eventually exit this world with a lot less body parts than when I entered. At last count, I'm minus two boobs, fourteen lymph nodes, a uterus, one cervix, two ovaries, and a couple of fallopian tubes. You gotta laugh, I mean, really. I still got my legs! If I don't keep a sense of humor I think it's all over. It's now fifteen years since I was first diagnosed, and I am ready for much more!

Anouk (San Francisco, California)

Surgical Treatments

Most patients with breast cancer have surgery to remove the cancer. These surgeries can have multiple effects for many women that have consequences beyond the realm of their cancer treatment.

Breast-conserving surgery aims to remove the cancer and some normal tissue around it but not the breast itself. Part of the chest wall lining may also be removed if the cancer is near it. This type of surgery may also be called lumpectomy, partial mastectomy, segmental mastectomy, or breast-sparing surgery.

Total mastectomy removes the entire breast that has cancer. This is also called a simple mastectomy. Some lymph nodes may also be removed and checked for cancer.

Modified radical mastectomy involves removing the whole breast that has cancer, many of the lymph nodes under the arm, the lining over the chest muscles, and, in some cases, part of the chest wall muscles.

For more information about surgical treatment for breast cancer, see Chapter 4.

—————————— **MY JOURNEY** ——————————

I was thirty-five years old when my doctor told me, "Debbie, you're young. We can do a partial mastectomy. Pardon me, but you're a large-breasted woman, so this type of surgery may help you in the long run, but what's important now is we can eliminate the cancer." I know he had good intentions, and he was right. I had big boobs, really big. I had plenty to spare. Two weeks later, I walked out of the hospital two sizes smaller. It took me quite a few days to adjust and regain my balance. I basically had to learn how to stand and walk all over again, as if I were a young teenager just starting to become a woman.

Debbie (Warren, Ohio)

Before and After Surgery

Chemotherapy may be given before surgery to shrink the tumor and reduce the amount of tissue that needs to be removed during the operation. Even if the surgeon removes all the cancer that is visible at the time of the surgery, some patients may be given radiation therapy, chemotherapy, or hormone therapy after surgery to kill any cancer cells that are left. Treatments given after the surgery to lower the risk that the cancer will come back are called adjuvant therapy.

Radiation Therapy (XRT)

This cancer treatment uses high-energy X-rays or other types of radiation to kill cancer cells or keep them from growing. Radiation therapy varies depending on the type and stage of the cancer being treated.

The following are two types of radiation therapy:

- *External* radiation uses a machine outside the body to send radiation toward the cancer.

- *Internal* radiation uses a radioactive substance sealed in needles, seeds, wires, or catheters placed directly into or near the cancer.

Chemotherapy

This treatment uses drugs to stop the growth of cancer cells, either by killing the cells or by stopping them from dividing. Traditional chemotherapies can have serious side effects because they tend to kill all rapidly dividing cells (like hair cells) somewhat indiscriminately.

Systemic chemotherapy is the administration of drugs that circulate throughout the entire body. Some systemic drugs are given by mouth, while others are infused into a vein or injected into a muscle. Systemic chemotherapy is used in the treatment of breast cancer.

Regional chemotherapy refers to drugs administered to only one area of the body, such as the cavity (peritoneum) surrounding the abdominal organs or the fluid (cerebrospinal fluid) that bathes the spinal cord and brain.

Chemotherapy options depend on the type of drug and the stage of cancer being treated.

Regimens

Consider the following example of three chemotherapy regimens that are commonly used to treat triple-negative breast cancer (TNBC).

One classical regimen used to treat TNBC is referred to as CMF, which are the initials of the three drugs used: cyclophosphamide, methotrexate, and 5-fluorouracil.

Another common regimen is FAC, which stands for 5-fluorouracil, anthracycline (daunorubicin), and cyclophosphamide.

These drug regimens are given intravenously.

For more information on specific drugs, we recommend the U.S. National Library of Medicine website.[5]

---

5. *http://dailymed.nlm.nih.gov/dailymed/*

In the near future, a targeted oral medication may become available to treat TNBC. This drug is called olaparib (Lynparza) and is currently approved by the FDA to treat hereditary breast cancer (Chapter 3).

Hormone Therapy

This cancer treatment removes hormones or blocks their action and stops cancer cells from growing. Hormones are substances made by glands in the body and circulated in the bloodstream, and some can cause certain cancers to grow.

If laboratory tests show that the cancer cells have places (receptors) where hormones can attach, then drugs can be given to block these receptors from working.

The ovaries are the main producer of estrogen, the hormone that makes some breast cancers grow. Treatment to stop the ovaries from making estrogen is called ovarian ablation and can be accomplished by surgery (removing the ovaries) or through using drugs.

Hormone therapy with tamoxifen (an antiestrogen) is often administered to patients with early, localized breast cancer that can be removed by surgery. It is also used for those with metastatic breast cancer that has spread to other parts of the body.

Tamoxifen or similar drugs can act on cells throughout the body and may increase the chance of developing endometrial cancer. Women taking tamoxifen should have a pelvic exam every year to look for any signs of cancer.

The following drugs work by blocking ER—the estrogen receptor:

- Fulvestrant (Faslodex)
- Raloxifene (Evista)
- Tamoxifen (Nolvadex)
- Toremifene (Fareston)

These drugs work by blocking the body's ability to make estrogen:

- Anastrozole (Arimidex)
- Exemestane (Aromasin)
- Letrozole (Femara)

For more information, we recommend the U.S. National Library of Medicine website.[6]

Cell-to-Cell Communication: Hormone and Growth Factor Receptors as Targets of Precision Medicines

For the specialized cells in our bodies to grow and function normally, they need to "talk" to or signal one another in ways that program or reprogram what they're doing at particular times. This cell-to-cell communication is carried out by a diverse variety of substances, such as hormones, like estrogen, and growth factors that bind to specific receptors on the surfaces of cells—like locks and keys that operate on-off switches.

Both hormones and growth factors signal cells to turn on or turn off certain functions, like milk production in the breast. Mutations in genes that cause cancer often act by corrupting these signaling systems, which result in uncontrolled cell growth and allow them to spread to other parts of the body (metastasize).

For example, HER2 is a growth-factor receptor that in small amounts is necessary to maintain the health of normal breast cells. However, in HER2+ breast cancer, abnormally large amounts of HER2 are produced on the outside of cells and this drives tumor growth.

---

6. http://dailymed.nlm.nih.gov/dailymed/

Targeted Therapy

Like a smart bomb, this type of treatment uses drugs to attack specific cancer cells with minimal or manageable side effects on normal cells. As we explained in Chapter 1, the drug imatinib (Gleevec) was a first-in-class drug of this kind, developed to treat a specific blood cancer. In the years since imatinib was developed, the same principles have led to a new generation of drugs that are used to treat a variety of solid tumors, such as lung cancer and breast cancer.

These targeted (precision medicine) drugs come in two forms:

1. *Small molecule drugs* come in pill form or as capsules to be taken orally. They are often labeled with the suffix "ib" or "nib." These drugs block certain cancer pathways inside cancer cells. One such drug used to treat HER2+ breast cancer is lapatinib (Tykerb). Another is palbociclib (Ibrance).
2. *Monoclonal antibody drugs,* sometimes called biologics, come as liquids that are injected into the body. These drugs are labeled with the suffix "mab." They work by binding to and blocking the action of receptors on the surfaces of cancer cells.

The following mab drugs are used to treat HER2+ breast cancer:

- Trastuzumab (Herceptin)
- Pertuzumab (Perjeta)
- Ado-trastuzumab emtansine (Kadcyla), a variation of trastuzumab, which is chemically combined with a small molecule drug. This arrangement is known as an antibody-drug conjugate.

For more information, we recommend the U.S. National Library of Medicine website.[7]

---

7. *http://dailymed.nlm.nih.gov/dailymed/*

Immunotherapy

Options are on the horizon for treating cancer by supporting our bodies' natural defenses and immune system. As described in Chapter 14, some of these options have already led to next-generation treatments for several types of cancer. At the present time, there are no FDA-approved immunotherapies for breast cancer, but research into this approach may soon yield breakthroughs in the treatment of breast cancer as it has for other cancer types.

Side Effects of Breast Cancer Treatment

After a mastectomy, the skin of the chest may feel tight. The surrounding muscles may feel stiff or weak. If muscles have been removed, other muscles will need to learn to take over for the missing muscles.

Two other potential postmastectomy complications involve the abnormal collection of fluid: seroma and lymphedema.

Seroma is a collection of serous fluid in the body where tissue has been removed by surgery. This sterile, clear to pale yellow body fluid

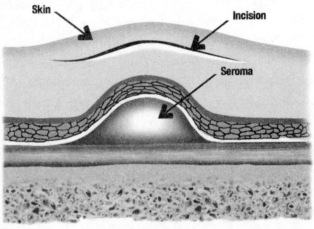

Seroma

lines the inside of body cavities. Fluid can build up under the skin close to an incision site. Seromas typically occur within one to two weeks after surgery. If the fluid builds up too much, the area will look swollen and may be painful.

If the seroma is small, nothing may need to be done. The body will reabsorb the excess fluid. Larger seromas are treated with removal of the excess fluid with a needle and syringe. This may need to be done more than once. Pain medication, such as acetaminophen or ibuprofen, may be suggested to aid with pain.

Although uncommon, seromas can become infected, so you should look out for signs of infection, including redness or warmth at the site and fever over 101.4 F, or drainage of cloudy or bloody fluid from the incision.

Lymphedema is the buildup of fluid in soft body tissue when the lymph system is damaged or blocked. It is a common problem that may be caused by cancer and cancer treatment. Lymphedema usually affects an arm or leg, but it can also affect other parts of the body.

Lymphedema can occur after any cancer or treatment that affects the flow of lymph through the lymph nodes, such as the removal of lymph nodes or radiation therapy. Lymphedema often occurs in breast cancer patients who have had all or part of the breast removed and axillary (underarm) lymph nodes removed.

Lymphedema may develop within days or it can occur many years after treatment. Most often it develops within three years of surgery.

Possible signs of lymphedema include the following:

- Swelling of an arm or leg, which may include fingers and toes
- A full or heavy feeling in an arm or leg
- A tight feeling in the skin
- Trouble moving a joint in the arm or leg

Normal

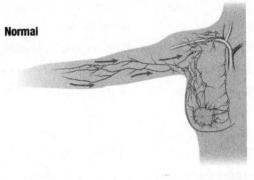

Lymphedema

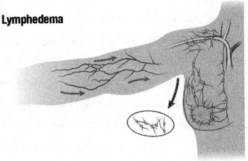

© Alila Medical Media – www.AlilaMedicalMedia.com

Lymphedema

- Thickening of the skin, with or without skin changes, such as blisters or warts
- A feeling of tightness when wearing clothing, shoes, bracelets, watches, or rings
- Itching or burning feeling in the legs or toes
- Trouble sleeping

Radiation therapy aimed at the chest may also cause the following side effects:

- Difficulty swallowing
- Shortness of breath

- Breast or nipple soreness
- Shoulder stiffness
- Cough, fever, and fullness of the chest, which is called radiation pneumonitis and usually happens two weeks to six months after radiation therapy.

—————————— MY JOURNEY ——————————

After my surgery and subsequent treatment, I was self-conscious from losing my hair and the swelling of my legs. Eventually, I managed to persuade myself that I was still me, no matter what I looked like. But I wasn't convinced until one day, while slumped over a cup of tea at an outdoor café, with a hat on my head and wearing long pants, a total stranger looked past my hairless head and pudgy ankles and told me I was beautiful. She said I reminded her of what real strength looks like, and that I must have a lot to live for, which I do! From then on, I not only started to manage the side effects much better, I actually took off my hat and started wearing shorts again.

Jane (Biloxi, Mississippi)

KEY POINTS TO REMEMBER

✓ The main person responsible for your health is you.

✓ Breast cancer is the second most common cancer in women after skin cancer.

✓ Be sure to let your doctors know if cancer of any type seems to run on either side of your family.

✓ If you were diagnosed with breast cancer before age fifty, or with triple-negative cancer before age sixty, or are of Jewish ancestry, ask to see a certified genetic counselor.

✓ A mammogram is an X-ray image of the breast and is a recommended screening tool for the early detection of breast cancer.

✓ Know your pathologist and the critical role she or he plays in your diagnosis and treatment.

✓ If you are asked to sign a consent form for a biopsy or other type of cancer surgery, ask whether there are any special protocols for processing your tissue based on the type of cancer you are suspected of having, and what tests will be performed on it.

✓ There are three main types of breast cancer and different medical treatments for each.

✓ DCIS is a stage 0 cancer that many doctors don't think should be called cancer at all.

✓ Immunotherapy is the latest breakthrough in cancer treatment but is not yet approved to treat breast cancer.

✓ Early diagnosis is key.

My New Besties

I was always someone who felt she could handle anything.
Throw it at me!
I'll handle it.
Then I was diagnosed.
"Oh, get a support group," my friend said.
"You need a whole group thing," said another.
"Shhhhhh," I said. "I'm fine."
Not!
Soon I realized what "alone" really meant.
Soon I realized what I needed.
Soon I craved information and the chance to relate to someone who "gets it."
Peer support.
My new besties . . .
Smartest thing I ever did.

—Anonymous

3

THE EXCEPTION, NOT THE RULE: Hereditary Breast Cancer and the Angelina Effect

I've always thought of myself as being a warrior.
When you actually have a battle,
it's better than when you don't know who to fight.

—Carly Simon, as told to *dailynews.com*

Two of the Most Famous Genes in the World

In 1994, after a decades-long international race, the mystery of why women in multiple generations of some families seemed doomed to develop breast and ovarian cancers was solved. Genetic research by investigators Mary-Claire King, PhD, and Mark Skolnick, PhD, isolated the first gene associated with hereditary breast cancer—the breast cancer 1 gene, or BRCA1. The National Cancer Institute of the National Institutes of Health supported this research.

Dr. James Watson, winner of the Nobel Prize for discovering the structure of DNA, said of this race, "There was no more exciting story in medical science."

Nineteen years later, in 2013, BRCA1 became famous on an entirely new level when actress and activist Angelina Jolie-Pitt announced that she had undergone surgery to remove both of her breasts because she had inherited a defective (mutant) copy of BRCA1 from her mother and grandmother. *Without* the surgery, she had up to an 87 percent chance of developing breast cancer.

In 1995, a team of British scientists successfully cloned a second gene, BRCA2, the cause of breast cancer in certain unfortunate families. Together, BRCA1 and BRCA2 launched a new era in breast and ovarian cancer prevention using the DNA of these genes to predict who was at the highest risk of developing these tumors.

All of this research and discovery has led to an entirely new set of questions:

- What exactly are these BRCA genes, and how do they cause cancer?
- Should every woman be tested?
- Are there any other options besides prophylactic surgery to remove a woman's breasts and/or ovaries to prevent cancer?

Founders and Carriers and Pedigrees—Oh My!

Everyone's DNA—a woman's *and* a man's—contains these two genes. So do dogs and cats, mice and rats, monkeys and all other mammals.

So why don't all of these creatures get cancer? Because BRCA1 and BRCA2 perform critical functions in normal cells that put the brakes on tumor formation by protecting us from environmental damage to our DNA. It's only when certain mutations deactivate or cripple these genes from performing their normal DNA repair functions that this leads to mutations in other oncogenes that cause cancer. Therefore, scientists refer to normal BRCA1 and BRCA2 genes as tumor suppressors.

In certain families, an ancestor suffered a DNA mutation in a BRCA1 or BRCA2 gene in their germ cells (eggs or sperm) and thereafter had a fifty-fifty chance of passing along the mutant gene to their daughters or sons. Such ancestors are called founders of the genetic mutation that then is passed along to many of their descendants across the generations. Descendants who inherit a defective copy of such a gene are called carriers. Medical infographics of family trees are called pedigrees and *must* be part of your personal health record.

The Angelina Effect

We will soon discover while examining Ms. Jolie's case in detail how it illustrates these concepts and how her example may or may not apply to you. Her public battle with hereditary breast and ovarian cancer—and the publicity surrounding it—created what we call the Angelina Effect, a dramatic increase in the number of women seeking genetic testing.

Sometimes, however, the differences between hereditary breast cancer and sporadic breast cancer (Chapter 2) have been misunderstood, leading to unnecessary and expensive testing and even false senses of security from negative results.

Actually, approximately 90 percent of us have normal BRCA1 and BRCA2 genes and they are doing their expected job, which is suppressing tumors. This doesn't mean you can't get breast cancer or ovarian cancer (Chapter 6); it's just that your risk is far lower than Ms. Jolie's and other people from families like hers with similar genetic profiles.

—————————— MY JOURNEY ——————————

Growing up in a time when many of us can gain access to our respective family trees, it should have come as no surprise when my daughters asked me one day about the history of cancer in our family. My girls had been searching online and had figured out that their grandmother, two of her sisters, two other aunts, and four cousins had all been stricken with cancer, and that there must be some connection. Was there something in the water?

I had no reason to get checked other than this trail of disease that has plagued our family. No symptoms. No reason to delve into something no one ever wants to discover, except for my daughters urging me to get checked. And I was too young! So I was floored when I gave in and had routine tests, which led to diagnostic mammograms and then a biopsy, which confirmed yet another case of cancer in our family.

Luckily, thanks to my girls, my breast cancer was detected early and I made it through without losing any body parts. During my treatment, I felt obliged to dig into our family history through a series of genetic tests with the hope of finding some reason why so many people in our family had gotten this nasty disease. Was there a link?

It was simple enough to figure out once my aunt was discovered to have the BRCA2 gene. The lab traced the gene back through our family tree and explained how the risk is multiplied and passed on from one generation to another. So one by one, we all got tested, and now, at least, each of us, with the gene or not, know our situation and can act accordingly. For me, it means considering possible preventative measures early enough in my life to make a difference. I have my girls to thank for that.

Camille (Chicago, Illinois)

The Family History of Marcheline Bertrand

Marcia Lynne ("Marcheline") Bertrand was born on May 9, 1950, at St. Francis Hospital in Blue Island, Illinois, a small town twenty miles south of downtown Chicago. Her father, Roland F. Bertrand, was of French-Canadian descent. Marcheline's mother was Lois June Gouwens of Dutch and German ancestry. After Marcheline, Roland and Lois June welcomed two other children. Debra was born in 1952, followed by their brother, Raleigh, a few years later.

In 1965, the family moved to Los Angeles, California, where Marcheline attended Beverly Hills High School. Her interest in acting flourished when she had the opportunity to study with the legendary acting teacher Lee Strasberg. This led to her landing a role in a TV series in 1971. That same year, she married actor Jon Voight. Both great joy and sorrow came into their lives in 1973 when she and Jon welcomed a son, James Haven, into the world, and soon after were forced to say good-bye to Marcheline's mother, Lois June Bertrand, who died from ovarian cancer at the young age of forty-five.

Two years later, in 1975, Marcheline and Jon had another child, whom they named Angelina Jolie. Undoubtedly influenced by their parents' acting vocations, both James and Angelina entered the film business. James became an actor and producer. Angelina, who began her career in 1991 at age sixteen, became an actor, director, writer, and producer. Over the following two decades, she went on to win numerous awards and became one of Hollywood's highest-paid actresses.

In 1999, the year Angelina won her first Golden Globe Award, her mother, Marcheline, was diagnosed with ovarian cancer. She eventually passed away from the disease in 2007 at the age of fifty-six. In 2004, Marcheline's sister and Angelina's aunt, Debbie, was diagnosed with breast cancer. She passed away nine years later at the age of sixty-one.

Marcheline had lived long enough to witness the birth of her first grandchild in 2006. At the age of thirty-one, Angelina Jolie added to her family of adopted children when she gave birth to a daughter, Shiloh Nouvel, whose father was Angelina's partner, Brad Pitt. They produced two other biological children in 2008, the fraternal twins Vivienne Marcheline and Knox Leon.

The Medical History of Angelina Jolie

How would a doctor or genetic counselor summarize Angelina's medical history in an infographic that would help to estimate her risk of breast and ovarian cancer? They would draw a pedigree diagram containing the key information.

The symbols in pedigree diagrams have special meanings. A square indicates a man, a circle stands for a woman, and a horizontal line connecting them indicates a marriage or other relationship resulting in children. If a person has a disease or other medical condition (in this case, cancer) their symbol is filled in. A long, slanted line through a square or circle indicates that the person has passed away. An arrow pointing to one of the symbols (Angelina in this case) means that person is the starting point for the genetic study of the family.

The pedigree shown here is a four-generation family history, beginning with Roland Bertrand and his wife, Lois June, and extending down to their three great-grandchildren, Shiloh and the twins, Vivienne and Knox.

Based on analysis of a diagram like this, Angelina's doctors recommended that her DNA be tested for abnormal copies of the BRCA1 and BRCA2 genes. She turned out to have mutations in BRCA1, which increased her lifetime risk of getting breast cancer up to 87 percent. With this information in hand, and under the care of Dr. Kristi Funk at the Pink Lotus Breast Center in Los Angeles, California,

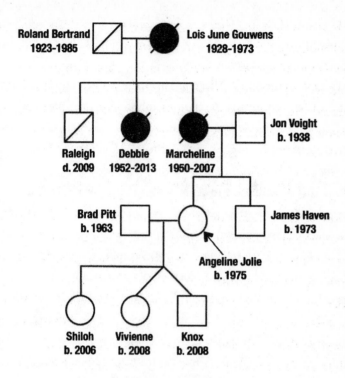

Pedigree Chart for Angelina Jolie-Pitt
Source: *CelebrityDiagnosis.com*

Ms. Jolie decided in 2013 to undergo prophylactic surgery, removing both of her breasts to prevent the possibility of ever getting breast cancer. Two years later, Angelina chose to have her ovaries removed as well because having a defective BRCA1 gene also gave her as great as a 60 percent chance of developing ovarian cancer (Chapter 6) in her lifetime.

Do I Have the Genes Like Angelina?

While very few of us can be like Angelina, if *any* kind of cancer (not just breast or ovarian) seems to run on either side of your family, ask your primary care physician or a gynecologist for a referral to a certified genetic counselor.

Before your meeting, collect and organize your family health information, as we did for the Bertrand family, and draw your own family tree. The U.S. Surgeon General's website helps people create a family health portrait that organizes the information *(https://familyhistory .hhs.gov/FHH/html/index.html)*.

Take this information to your doctor's appointment. Since many doctors are not experts in genetics, don't be afraid to ask for a referral to a cancer genetic counselor. Most hospitals that have cancer centers will have genetic counselors on staff. If you have trouble finding one, you can always get in touch with the National Society of Genetic Counselors *(www.nsgc.org/)* and ask for help in locating a qualified counselor near you. There are also companies that offer counseling services online or by phone *(http://www/mygenecounsel.com)*. A genetic counselor will review your family health history data and offer a recommendation about whether or not you should have your DNA tested.

A large survey called EMBRACE (Epidemiological Study of Familial Breast Cancer), published in 2013,[8] may provide the best estimates for cancer risk in women who carry abnormal copies of the BRCA1 or BRCA2 genes. If your BRCA1 or BRCA2 genes are abnormal, that is, the test is positive, EMBRACE says this about your risk of developing cancer: "BRCA1 mutation carriers have a 60 percent risk of developing breast cancer by age 70 and a 59 percent chance of developing ovarian cancer. BRCA2 mutation carriers have a 55 percent risk of developing breast cancer by age 70 and a 16.5 percent chance of developing ovarian cancer."

---

8. *http://ccge.medschl.cam.ac.uk/embrace/*

If you undergo testing and your BRCA1 and BRCA2 genes are normal, that is, the test is negative, this doesn't mean that you won't ever develop breast cancer. In fact, according to the National Cancer Institute, you'll still have about a one in eight (12.4 percent) chance of developing breast cancer in your lifetime (Chapter 2). You should still have regular checkups and screening tests (Chapter 13) as recommended by your doctor.

It's important to understand that these risk numbers are averages for American women. Your personal risks may be higher or lower depending on your medical history as well as environmental or lifestyle factors. A cancer genetic counselor will be able to personalize your risk based on the risk model that best applies to you.

I'm at Risk—What Do I Do?

Once your doctor receives your genetic counselor's report, it's time to consider how you want to manage your personal risks. You have basically three options.

1. *"Watchful waiting" or surveillance.* This means your healthcare provider will use the usual methods of screening for breast cancer (exams, mammography) but will employ them more frequently. Screening for ovarian cancer is done using transvaginal ultrasound imaging and also periodically measuring a chemical in your blood called CA-125. Angelina Jolie used watchful waiting for the two years between her breast surgery in 2013 and the removal of her ovaries in 2015. She decided to have her ovaries removed because her levels of CA-125 began to rise.

2. *Risk-reducing surgery (prophylactic mastectomy).* Removing the breasts reduces the possibility of developing breast cancer

by 90 percent but does not completely eliminate it. Removal of the ovaries and fallopian tubes (bilateral salpingo-oophorectomy) eliminates the risk of cancer but also causes forced menopause and is usually recommended for women only after they no longer want any new children.

3. *Chemoprevention (pharmacoprevention).* This involves using drugs like Tamoxifen (an antiestrogen) and is controversial because most genetic breast cancers are triple-negative cancers that are not estrogen-sensitive (Chapter 2).

Before you commit to any of these options, ask to be connected with other women who have faced the same risks as you and talk to them about their decision process.

> **NOTE to PATIENT:**
> Never be afraid to get a second professional opinion.

Committing to a specific course of action or treatment plan is an enormous decision, and we recommend you do your due diligence beforehand. If you do have a cancer gene like BRCA1 in your DNA, a cancer is not going to develop overnight. You have plenty of time to carefully investigate and consider all of your options so that you can make the most informed choice possible. Remember, Angelina waited two years before making the decision to have her ovaries removed.

I've Got Breast Cancer—Now What?

Breast cancers that develop in BRCA1 carriers are often the triple-negative type and are treated the same way as in noncarrier women (Chapter 2). The main difference is that women with BRCA1 or BRCA2 mutations and a cancer in one breast have up to a 60 percent chance of developing cancer in the other breast within ten years and need to consider either watchful waiting or preventive surgery.

———————————— MY JOURNEY ————————————

There's nothing you can do about it if you get hit by a bus you didn't see coming. But if you see the bus and try to cross the street anyway, you're not playing the odds very well. It's the same thing with cancer. Prevention is key.

For women under forty—who as a group are not yet recommended to have mammograms—I suggest you add this to your general health protocol if you have *any* history of cancer—especially breast cancer—in your family. Way too many women get diagnosed too late because they had no symptoms or reason to check. With science progressing as it is, doctors can trace family history much better and determine if you are a good candidate for early testing.

Some "crazy" hunch led me to get tested when I was only thirty-five, and it ended up saving my life. I hope women with any family trail of cancer will follow my example.

Suzanne (Pittsburgh, Pennsylvania)

Beyond the BRCA Gene— Other Family Syndromes

BRCA1 and BRCA2 are not the only genes associated with cancers that run in families. Following are other sample syndromes and the genes responsible for them.

1. *Li-Fraumeni syndrome.* In this case, mutations are in a gene called TP53. Many other cancers besides breast cancer can

develop in these patients at unusually young ages. Patients
with Li-Fraumeni have a 21 to 49 percent chance of developing a cancer by the age of thirty and carry a 68 to 93 percent
risk of developing a cancer in their lifetimes.

2. *Cowden syndrome.* This is caused by abnormalities in a gene
called PTEN. Women with Cowden syndrome have a 25 to
50 percent risk of cancer in their lifetimes, and these cancers
tend to occur at a young age.

3. *Peutz-Jeghers syndrome.* Mutation in a gene called STK11
causes this, and women affected by this disease are fifteen
times more likely to develop breast cancer than the average
woman.

All three of these conditions are quite rare. It's the job of genetic
counselors to diagnose these conditions based on your medical and
family history, recommend further testing, and, if necessary, refer you
to the right specialists for treatment.

What About Men with BRCA Genes?

Contrary to popular belief, men with BRCA1 and BRCA2 genes
do get breast cancer, just not as frequently as women. This is simply
because of biology. Men don't have as much breast tissue as women,
and their bodies don't experience the same hormonal (estrogen) cycles
as women do during their reproductive years. For men with BRCA1
mutations, the lifetime risk of developing breast cancer is only 1 to 5
percent compared with up to 87 percent in women. The lifetime risk
numbers for BRCA2 mutations are a bit higher among men at 5 to
10 percent.

Genetic Progress and the Future

Mary-Claire King, professor of genome sciences and of medicine at the University of Washington, discovered the region on the genome that eventually became known as BRCA1. King told Alice Park of *Time*[9] in 2014, "If we cast our minds back to the 1970s, when my work [on BRCA] began, the mainstream theory was that breast cancer was viral. And some cancers are, so it wasn't a crazy theory. My thinking—and, believe me, this was not a theory in the field but just a notion I had—was that there was good evidence that there were some families in which breast cancer was especially common. There was no evidence of a smoking gun. That opened the possibility that there was something else. That went side by side in my mind with the logical way of thinking about cancer, that all cancer is genetic in the sense that it's a consequence of changes in DNA. That also was not mainstream thinking at the time."

And as time changes and progress continues, we see that cancer, through the lens of pathology and other science, is being reconsidered. Nearly fifty years ago, when King and her colleagues first explored this aspect of genomic science, they never imagined that within a few decades oncologists and medical geneticists would be able to take what King and others had developed and use it to invent the capability for testing women (and men) to decipher if mutations were present, and, as a result of these findings, to save lives!

Imagine what science will uncover in the next few decades. We have devoted researchers, generous celebrities, and courageous patients participating in testing trials to thank for all of this progress.

---

9. *http://time.com/2802156/lessons-from-the-woman-who-discovered-the-brca-cancer-gene/*

KEY POINTS TO REMEMBER

✓ Most of breast cancers (about 90 percent) do not run
   in families and are *not* caused by faulty BRCA1 or
   BRCA2 genes.

✓ If your BRCA1 test is positive for mutations in the gene,
   you have up to an 85 percent chance of developing
   breast cancer by age 70 and a 59 percent chance of
   developing ovarian cancer (Chapter 6).

✓ If your BRCA2 test is positive, you have an 80 percent
   chance of developing breast cancer by age seventy
   and a 50 percent chance of developing ovarian cancer
   (Chapter 6).

✓ Other genes besides BRCA1 and BRCA2 can cause
   breast cancers that run in families.

✓ A genetic counselor can help you figure out your
   unique situation and risks.

✓ Men get hereditary breast cancer, too, but less often
   than women.

HIGH RISK

I can't decide.
Ugh.
I'm a Libra. Is that my curse?
Scales, scales, always scales,
weighing every decision as if it's my last.

I tested positive for the BRCA1 gene mutation.
I was thirty-three!

Wait. Where's the information? What do I do?
Where are those risk-management tutorials when you need them?

They're throwing numbers at me right and left.
I'm up 68 percent on this and down 34 percent on that.

If I do this, that might happen.
If I do that, we're not sure, but maybe this or maybe that.

No big history in my family, so what's a girl to do?
I need a plan. Yes, a plan would be good.
They're encouraging me to have a plan.

I'm at risk.
This is America, home of the best X-ray machines in the world.
Let's lay low and keep checking every now and then.
How's that?
I don't have cancer (yet).
My breasts, do I need them? Are you sure?
But what if it doesn't come?
What if?

—Maze Beck

4 BREAST CANCER SURGERY: What's Right for You?

I'm stronger than I thought I was.
My favorite phrase has been "This too shall pass."
I now understand it really well.

—**Robin Roberts**, as told to *Parade*

When Surviving Becomes Thriving

For many years the focus of breast cancer treatment has been solely aimed at patient survival. Now, as survival rates continue to improve, quality of life *after* cancer has become an equally important aspect of caring for patients.

Breast reconstruction has therefore become a key consideration in any treatment plan.

We will discuss specific types of breast reconstruction in Chapter 5, but increasingly more often, reconstruction is started or done simultaneously with the surgical treatments described in this chapter.

――――――――――― MY JOURNEY ―――――――――――

As my anesthesiologist was getting ready to knock me out for surgery, he told me I was looking good, that I was as healthy as can be and had nothing to worry about. I looked up from the gurney at him and said, "You must be joking."

He said, "Oh no, you're great, except for the breast cancer."

Angela (Dallas, Texas)

Martina Navratilova: The Legend Lives On!

On February 24, 2010, women's tennis great Martina Navratilova received news from her physician. "'Your biopsies are positive,' I was told. I was, like, 'Positive is usually good, but wait a minute, that is not good; what does it mean?'"

For the nine-time Wimbledon singles champion who holds more singles and doubles titles than anyone in history, it meant that the lump detected during a routine mammogram a month earlier was cancerous. Her diagnosis, called ductal carcinoma *in situ* (DCIS), is, fortunately, a common form of noninvasive cancer, sometimes referred to as stage 0 breast cancer, or precancerous, as described in Chapter 2.

Navratilova underwent a lumpectomy. Less than two weeks after the surgery, she competed in the twenty-five-mile cycling portion of a triathlon in Hawaii.

To decrease the chance of the cancer returning, Navratilova had radiation therapy four times a week for six weeks. She received her treatments in Paris so she could still practice for the 2010 French Open. Although she was feeling some side effects (soreness and fatigue) from the radiation therapy, she and partner Jana Novotná easily won the Women's Legends Doubles. Once again, Navratilova proved to be an inspiration for many.

Different Types of Surgery

Depending on your specific condition and a plethora of other factors, you may have several options regarding which type of surgery is right for you. These include four different categories, presented here:

Breast-Conserving Procedures

Most women with early-stage breast cancer will be eligible for breast-conserving surgery (BCS), a procedure designed to remove cancer from the breast and some normal tissue around it but not the breast itself. This surgery is referred to by a number of names, including lumpectomy, partial mastectomy, and segmental mastectomy.

A special type of breast-conserving surgery is called conservative mastectomy and usually means that your surgical team will remove the cancer using plastic surgery techniques that preserve your nipple and much of your skin.

Angelina Jolie's doctors used an approach like this (Chapter 5). But it must be noted that Ms. Jolie didn't actually have cancer at the time, and based on her genetic risk (Chapter 3), she chose to have a double mastectomy to prevent cancer.

Nevertheless, many women with breast cancer can also be treated with oncoplastic techniques (Chapter 5), although these are more difficult to perform than traditional lumpectomies and simple mastectomies.

Typically, women who undergo breast-conserving surgery also need to follow up with a course of radiation therapy, which is usually five days a week for five to eight weeks.

After the procedure, your breast may look similar to its original appearance. However, if the tumor is large, it may look different. There may be a loss of volume in the area of the scar, and these may be able to be filled in later with fat grafts (Chapter 5).

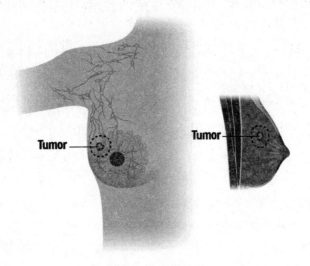

Breast Conserving Surgery
Source: © Alila Medical Media—*www.AlilaMedicalMedia.com*

You should still have feeling in your breast, nipple, and areola. Most women will have some pain after the procedure, but women who undergo BCS are ready to return to their usual range of activities within five to ten days.

Studies have shown that for women who have the option, lumpectomy plus radiation therapy is just as effective as mastectomy for treating early breast cancer. These studies looked at the overall survival rate of women treated with either option. Overall survival refers to the percentage of people remaining alive for a certain period of time after the diagnosis of a disease, such as breast cancer, or treatment for a disease.

What is the chance that the cancer will come back?

Approximately 10 percent of women who have BCS plus radiation therapy will be diagnosed with a second cancer in the same breast within twelve years of the first procedure. If your cancer does return, it is unlikely to affect how long you live.

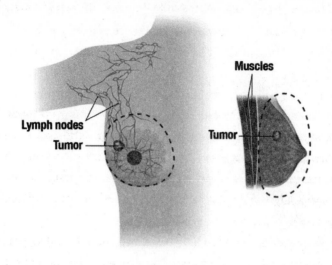

Total Mastectomy
Source: © Alila Medical Media—*www.AlilaMedicalMedia.com*

For some women, preoperative treatment, called neoadjuvant therapy, may shrink a tumor sufficiently so that a lumpectomy may then become an option.

Total or Simple Mastectomy

This surgery removes an entire breast that has cancer in it. This is also the type of surgery performed in women who have an increased risk of developing breast cancer because of their genes (Chapter 3).

During the procedure, your breast and nipple will be removed, unless oncoplastic techniques are used. You will have a flat chest on the side of your body where the breast has been removed. On average, it may take three to four weeks after a mastectomy to feel something approaching normal.

After surgery, the skin around where the surgeon cut, as well as the area under your arm, will be numb. This numbness usually improves over the next one to two years, although it may never feel completely like it used to. Some women, especially those with larger breasts, may feel out of balance after the procedure, which may lead to neck and shoulder pain.

There is a smaller chance that your cancer will return in the same area than if you have breast-conserving surgery. About 5 percent of women who have a mastectomy will get cancer on that same side of the chest within twelve years.

Modified Radical Mastectomy

This surgery removes an entire breast with cancer, along with many of the lymph nodes under the arm, the lining over the chest muscles, and, in some cases, part of the chest wall muscles. Patients with invasive breast cancer undergo modified radical mastectomies so that the lymph nodes can be examined, which helps to identify whether cancer cells may have spread beyond the breast.

Chemotherapy may be given before surgery to remove the tumor. When this happens, it will shrink the tumor and reduce the amount of tissue that needs to be removed during surgery. This type of treatment given before surgery is referred to as preoperative therapy, or neoadjuvant therapy.

Even if the doctor removes all the cancer that can be seen at the time of the surgery, some patients may receive radiation therapy, chemotherapy, or hormone therapy after surgery, which aims to kill any remaining microscopic areas of cancer cells. Treatment received after the surgery, to lower the risk that the cancer will come back, is called adjuvant or postoperative therapy.

Lymph Node Surgery

During any of the aforementioned procedures, the physician will also remove a lymph node, known as the sentinel lymph node. As the

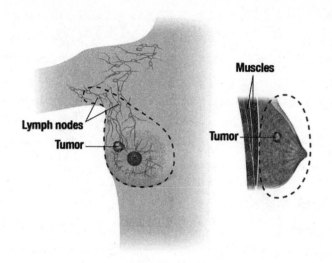

Modified Radical Mastectomy
Source: © Alila Medical Media—*www.AlilaMedicalMedia.com*

name implies, a sentinel is a guard, whose job it is to keep watch. This is the first lymph node to receive the lymphatic drainage from a tumor and the first through which cancer is likely to spread.

To perform a sentinel lymph node biopsy (SLNB), a radioactive substance/blue dye is injected near the tumor. It flows through the lymph ducts to the lymph nodes. The first lymph node to receive the substance or dye is removed. A pathologist views the tissue under a microscope to look for cancer cells.

Based on these results, the surgeon removes the tumor using breast-conserving surgery or mastectomy. If no cancer cells are found, it may not be necessary to remove any additional lymph nodes. On the other hand, if cancer cells are found, more lymph nodes will be removed through a separate incision. This is called a lymph node dissection.

Sentinel lymph node biopsies are useful for several reasons:

- To help doctors assign a stage to a patient's cancer (Chapter 1)

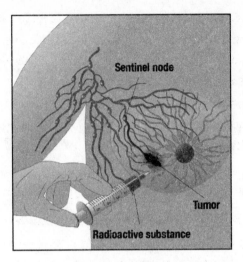

Sentinel Lymph Node Biopsy
Source: ellepigrafica

- To estimate the risk that tumor cells have developed the ability to spread to other parts of the body
- To allow some patients to avoid more extensive lymph node surgery

All lymph node surgery can have adverse effects, and some of these may be reduced or avoided if fewer lymph nodes are removed.

Potential adverse effects of lymph node surgery include the following:

- Lymphedema (tissue swelling)—During SLNB or more extensive lymph node surgery, lymph vessels leading to and from a group of nodes are cut, thereby disrupting the normal flow of lymph through the affected area. This disruption may lead to an abnormal buildup of lymph fluid. In addition to swelling, patients with lymphedema may experience pain or discomfort in the affected area, and the overlying skin may become thickened or hard. In the case of extensive lymph node surgery in an armpit or groin, the swelling may affect an entire arm or leg. In addition, there is an increased risk of infection in the affected area or limb.

- Seroma, the buildup of lymph fluid at the site of the surgery
- Numbness, tingling, or pain at the site of the surgery
- Difficulty moving the affected body part

Sharon Osbourne: A "No-Brainer" Decision

This larger-than-life personality has never been shy from telling things as they are. So it wasn't especially surprising when, in 2012, the matriarch of the Osbourne family (wife of heavy metal singer Ozzy Osbourne and mother of Jack and Kelly Osbourne) went public with the news that she had undergone a bilateral mastectomy.

In 2010, Sharon and Ozzy both had their genomes analyzed, and while Ozzy's came up clean, Sharon's revealed that she had both the colon cancer gene, for which she was treated in 2002, as well as the breast cancer gene. This prompted Sharon to have both breasts removed.

"As soon as I found out I had the breast cancer gene, I thought, *the odds are not in my favor*," she told the British magazine *Hello!* "I've had cancer before and I didn't want to live under that cloud. I decided to just take everything off and had a double mastectomy. For me, it wasn't a big decision; it was a no-brainer. I want to be around for a long time and be a grandmother to Pearl [daughter of her son Jack]."

Which Treatment Is Right for Me?

After your cancer diagnosis, you should have enough time to meet with breast cancer surgeons, learn about your surgery choices, and think about what is important to you. Learning as much as possible about your condition can help you make a choice you feel good about.

To make sure that happens, talk with a breast cancer surgeon about what happens during surgery, the types of problems that sometimes occur, and any treatment you might need after surgery. To get a better idea of what to expect, ask your surgeon if you can see before and after pictures of other women who have had different types of surgery.

Ask as many questions as possible. Talking to family members, friends, or others who have had surgery may also be useful. Locate other people with similar circumstances to yours by perusing several different websites devoted to helping patients and caregivers find online support and valuable information from those who have experienced many of the same things you are about to face.

Lillie Shockney, RN, who has worked for many years at Johns Hopkins Breast Cancer Center as an oncology nurse taking care of women with breast cancer (as well as having her own personal diagnosis in 1992 and 1994), has come to appreciate the importance of assessing a woman's feelings about her breasts before surgery. When first talking with a patient about her diagnosis and surgical treatment plan, she tries to learn about that individual woman's relationship with her breasts.

Shockney says, "Once a woman overcomes the immediate fear of losing her life, her next fear usually is losing part or all of her breast. It is important to understand how closely her perception of her body image and self-image is tied to her breasts. For many, the fear of how others will perceive her altered body image is also difficult."

Every woman who has been diagnosed with breast cancer ought to share her feelings about this with her surgical oncologist and oncology nurse. They need to know how their patient is handling this part of the process. At the end of the day, patient participation is key.

"Be sure the type of surgery you choose also addresses your psychological well-being," Shockney says. "We each have the right to choose after careful thought, education, and planning. A year after a woman completes her treatment, I want to hear her say, 'I'm happy with the treatment choices I made.'"

Committed healthcare providers *want* to know how their patients feel about their bodies, and in the case of women facing breast cancer surgery, where their appearance may be forever altered, it is especially crucial that this information be shared. For doctors and nurses, it can offer valuable insight into how well a woman is likely to cope with her upcoming surgery. This understanding can influence how treatment will eventually be administered.

It's a question of setting yourself up correctly to be treated as a whole person and not just a body experiencing a disease.

—————————— MY JOURNEY ——————————

When I found out I had breast cancer, the first thing I thought was, "No way. I'm not having my breast removed!" I wasn't about to lose either one of them. I didn't know if I wanted a lumpectomy, either. But that's what my doctor recommended, which didn't go down well with me.

What about doing nothing? Or, something like that?

After hashing through all of these options, I decided to go against the grain and skip *any* type of surgery. Instead, I opted for a regimen of drugs and a clinical trial to monitor my condition with mammograms and MRIs.

No surgery. No radiation. No chemo. So far, so good.

Hallie (Lansing, Michigan)

The Importance of Second Opinions

As we explained in Chapter 2, the doctor who actually diagnoses your cancer is your pathologist. Everyone else on your care team, including your surgeon, are planning treatment for you based on the report your pathologist has sent back from the lab. It's your right to see this report, and we strongly encourage you to do so.

Your case may even have been presented at your hospital's tumor board. Tumor boards are regular meetings during which cancer diagnoses and treatment plans are discussed. These meetings are attended by all of the specialists taking care of the patient, including the pathologist, medical oncologist, surgeon, etc., and they review cases to make sure that everyone is on the same page regarding the precise diagnosis and personalized treatment plan.

Although a pathologist's diagnosis is cut-and-dried most of the time, this is not always the case, as we saw in Rita Wilson's story in Chapter 2. If you have any doubt or uncertainty about the pathologist's diagnosis, seek an initial second opinion from another pathologist who is a specialist in your cancer type. She or he can make sure that the first pathologist's diagnosis was accurate and complete and that all of the appropriate DNA testing has been done on your biopsy specimen.

To learn more about what pathologists do and what roles they play in your care, visit the College of American Pathologists (CAP) at *www.cap.org*. Cancer surgeons work very closely with pathologists to ensure that each patient under their care receives the right diagnosis and the proper treatment.

Your surgeon will recommend a specific treatment plan for you. Since honest differences of opinion exist among surgeons about what is best for a patient, don't worry about hurting your doctor's feelings by asking for a second opinion. This practice is very common and, in fact, some insurance companies even require it.

The Gift

In her memoir and "how-to" book, *It's Just a Word: Reclaiming Your Life Through Cancer—Beautifully,*[10] which is part of *The Cancer Book: 101 Stories of Courage, Support and Love,* Elizabeth Bayer offers many practical tips for those facing surgery, as well as a spiritual compass we might all be wise to consider.

First, she advises you to preserve your energy by getting a friend or family member to serve as your team leader in order to remove the burden of having to keep everyone—friends, family, coworkers, lawyer, accountant, etc.—informed about your surgery, subsequent progress, etc. That person may also assist you in securing disability, if needed (even temporarily), as well as a host of other overwhelming administrative details requiring immediate attention.

When you provide your team leader with a list of VIPs, this will give you an opportunity to revisit who these people are and why they are so important in your life. This list can include the person charged with medical power of attorney (healthcare proxy), living will, and traditional will.

"Make sure you choose well when assigning medical power of attorney," Elizabeth says. "Doctors will not give out any information to anyone without a signed medical power of attorney/healthcare proxy. Saying you are next of kin means nothing without the document."

This can take time, so once surgery is scheduled, do not delay your preparations. If possible, allow enough time to get all of this settled and your team in place before the surgery. Peace of mind—for everyone concerned—is vital to your eventual healing.

Asking questions is essential. For Elizabeth, this meant asking better questions, ones that really made sense for her. "These questions

---

10. Chicken Soup for the Soul Publishing 2009, Copyright 2009 Chicken Soup for the Soul Publishing, LLC.

changed everything for me. And, even though many very experienced healers were indicating that I might not need surgery, I knew, deep down to the core of my being, that the gift *was* the surgery."

Questions to Ask About Reconstruction

If you think you might have a mastectomy, this is also a good time to learn about breast reconstruction. Consider meeting with a reconstructive plastic surgeon to learn about this surgery and if it seems like a good option for you. Think about what is important to *you*.

The following questions may help you decide what is most important:

- If I have breast-sparing surgery, am I willing and able to have radiation therapy five days a week for five to eight weeks?
- If I have a mastectomy, do I also want breast reconstruction surgery?
- If I have breast reconstruction surgery, do I want it at the same time as my mastectomy?
- What treatment does my insurance cover? What do I have to pay for?
- How important is it to me how my breast looks after cancer surgery?
- How important is it to me how my breast feels after cancer surgery?
- If I have a mastectomy and do not have reconstruction, will my insurance cover my prostheses and special bras?
- Where can I find breast prostheses and special bras?

Being well informed about the different options and deciding which factors are most important to you will allow you to make the best decision for yourself and your family.

Prosthetics as an Alternative to Reconstruction and Mastectomy-Friendly Clothing

With improvements in surgical techniques, breast reconstruction has becoming increasingly popular for breast cancer patients. However, not all women elect to undergo reconstruction. According to a 2014 article in the *Journal of Clinical Oncology*, 37 percent of women who have undergone a lumpectomy or mastectomy elect not to have reconstructive surgery.

The reasons for this are varied and include the following:

- Some women are less concerned about the changes in their bodies and feel reconstruction is not necessary for them.
- Some women do not wish to have any further surgical procedures or series of procedures necessary to get a good surgical result.
- There is a risk that the reconstruction will fail.
- There may be other medical reasons why surgery or anesthesia is not possible.
- They want additional time to make a decision about breast reconstruction.

For these women, the use of a breast prosthesis may be a good choice. This is an artificial breast form that can be worn after a mastectomy that replaces the shape of all or part of the breast that has been removed. Many women opt for this because they want to wear the same clothing they wore prior to the surgery. They also may want to look natural and symmetrical.

There are two general types of prosthesis:

1. *A lightweight model made of polyfill or foam.* This kind is often recommended when you are recovering from surgery.

It is most comfortable, especially against skin that may still
be irritated from surgery or radiation. It may also fare a little
better in warm weather and can be used while swimming.
One last plus—it is machine washable.

2. *A prosthesis made from silicone, a soft gel-like substance.*
This kind may look more realistic and feel more natural to
you for everyday wear.

Both types can be fit into a pocket in a specially designed bra (a post-
mastectomy bra) or camisole, which will hold the prosthesis in place.
Some silicone prostheses can be used without a bra, as they have adhe-
sive patches that attach to your breast area. The patches last about a week
before they need to be replaced. Other silicone prostheses have magnetic
strips that attach to your skin and to the breast form to hold it in place.

Prostheses come in a variety of shades designed to closely match
with your own skin tone. They also come in a variety of shapes:

- *Symmetrical:* This is usually an oval or triangular shape, which
can be worn on either the left or right side.
- *Teardrop:* This is often more suitable for women whose breasts
are fuller in the lower and outer area and less full above the
nipple. These can also be worn on the right or left side.
- *Asymmetrical:* These are generally more suitable for women
who have had more extensive surgery, as they have extensions
to fit under the arm or upper chest wall. They are specifically
designed for the left or right side.

Silicone breast prostheses are also considered weighted, meaning
that they are designed not only to simulate the shape, but the *weight*
of the missing breast tissue. Proponents of weighted breast forms say
that they restore balance, helping to keep your shoulders even and
your posture straight.

You can buy a breast prosthesis from many different sources, including surgical supply stores, pharmacies, or custom lingerie shops, which usually have certified fitters specifically trained to fit women for breast prostheses. Some even provide private service in your home. Ask your physician, oncology nurse, local American Cancer Society program, or other local breast cancer support groups for their recommendations for nearby breast prosthesis vendors.

This leads us to a crucial question: What does a breast prosthesis cost?

The prices vary greatly. Some fiberfill forms can cost as little as $10. Foam forms run about $30 to $70 or more. Prices range from under $100 to $500 for high-quality, weighted silicone forms. They usually last from two to five years. Silicone is hand washable only. It's important to note that salt or pool water, as well as hot tubs, may damage the outer shell of silicone products. They can become sticky, which can collect dirt, or thinner, which can lead to leaks or rupture.

Insurance coverage of breast prostheses vary greatly. Be sure to ask your doctor for a prescription for the prosthesis, as well as for post-mastectomy bras, and check with your insurance company before purchasing one.

A number of retail companies, such as Sears, Lands' End, and JC Penney, as well as online retailers and specialty shops, sell bathing suits and lingerie designed for women who have had mastectomies. The clothing comes with a pocket to hold the prosthesis. You can also sew pockets into the bras or clothing you already own.

Once again, whenever possible, we encourage you to speak directly with women who have already undergone the procedure you are considering and have experience with the prosthesis you may be eventually wearing. Only someone who has lived it can really tell you what it's like. When you do your due diligence, you will feel more relaxed and confident heading into your own adventure.

KEY POINTS TO REMEMBER

✓ Life *after* cancer has become an important aspect of caring for patients.

✓ Different kinds of surgery to treat breast cancer can be equally effective in curing or controlling the disease.

✓ Each patient has options that need to be fully explored. Your participation in the process is key.

✓ Talk with your doctor about what happens during surgery, the types of complications that sometimes occur, and whether or not you'll need additional treatment besides surgery.

✓ You can get a second opinion on what type of cancer you have from a pathologist and on your treatment and reconstruction options from another surgeon.

✓ Be sure the type of surgery you choose also addresses your cosmetic goals and psychological well-being.

✓ Mastectomy-friendly clothing and prostheses are available for women as alternatives to reconstructive surgery.

The Shower

Warm water probes my bald head,
where long hair used to diffuse
the chains of drops.

Savoring a moment of being alone,
I glance down to watch the water
leave my feet and run to the exit.

Strangely,
I see a clear view
of only one foot.

The other,
partly obstructed
by the intrusion of my breast.

Ah, yes.
Cancer.

—Laura L. Strebel

5 ONCOPLASTIC SURGERY AND BREAST RECONSTRUCTION: A Very Personal Journey

*I do not feel any less of a woman.
I feel empowered that I made a strong choice
that in no way diminishes my femininity.*

—Angelina Jolie-Pitt, from the *New York Times*

The Times They Are a-Changin'

Surgical treatment of breast cancer used to rely on radical, often disfiguring, procedures based on a more primitive and incomplete knowledge of cancer biology and decidedly less sophisticated surgical techniques than we have today. An increasing number of breast cancers are becoming curable because of better screening technologies that allow for early detection of tumors. As a result, cancer is being reimagined as a more manageable illness, and the goals of breast cancer surgery have broadened from a singular focus on eradicating the cancer to a dual focus that includes better cosmetic outcomes and improved quality of life for patients.

These changes in the philosophy of breast cancer surgery are so profound that they merit a new designation.

Oncoplastic surgery is a new interdisciplinary field that combines the latest esthetic plastic and reconstructive surgery techniques with the safe and effective practice of surgical oncology. For example, Los Angeles surgeon Dr. Joel Aronowitz, a prominent specialist in this new field, used another new technique—belly fat stem cell transplantation—to repair the breasts of actress Suzanne Somers more than ten years after they were damaged by her lumpectomy and radiation therapy for cancer in 2001. Dr. Aronowitz is a champion of nipple and skin-sparing "conservative mastectomies" and an advocate of surgical decision making that takes into account the personalized needs and unique anatomy of each patient. We'll present more about his work later in this chapter, but first it's apropos to describe some of the basics.

Finding Your Best Option:
How Christina Applegate and Angelina
Made Their Decisions

After a mastectomy, women have multiple options regarding common procedures for restoring, rebuilding, the shape of the breast or breasts removed during surgery. This is referred to as breast reconstruction.

Christina Applegate brought this subject to national attention when she appeared on the April 2009 cover of *People* magazine as one of America's *100 Most Beautiful People*. Fifteen months earlier,

Christina had undergone a double mastectomy with breast reconstruction. Although cancer was diagnosed in only one of her breasts, she opted to have them both removed because of a condition she shares with Angelina Jolie-Pitt: carrier of mutations in the BRCA1 gene (Chapter 3).

A woman's first option is for the surgeon to initiate the first stage in rebuilding the breast at the same time he or she performs the mastectomy.

If the patient chooses a second option by delaying reconstruction, the surgeon performs the initial stage of rebuilding the breast only after the chest has healed from the mastectomy and any necessary adjuvant therapy has been administered.

A third option is called immediate-delayed reconstruction. With this method, doctors use a tissue expander, a balloon-like structure that can be filled with salt water (saline) and placed under the skin during the mastectomy. The expander's job is to preserve space for an implant while the pathologist analyzes the cancerous tissue that has been removed to determine if the surgeon was able to remove the entire tumor. If not, the patient may need radiation therapy, so breast reconstruction may be delayed until this treatment is completed.

As discussed in Chapter 3, Angelina Jolie-Pitt was diagnosed as a carrier of BRCA1 gene mutations, putting her at high risk for developing breast cancer. Because of this, she decided to minimize her risk by undergoing a prophylactic bilateral mastectomy and breast reconstruction.

To raise awareness of hereditary breast cancer, Jolie-Pitt went public with her case with an op-ed article in the *New York Times* describing how she came to her decision and why women should not be afraid to discuss their options with their physicians.

Angelina not only explained her breast reconstruction procedure, she went further, giving permission to her surgeon, Dr. Kristi Funk, to describe in detail the medical information about her case and the stages of treatment she underwent. (This information is contained in a blog called "A Patient's Journey: Angelina Jolie" at *PinkLotusBreastCenter .com.*)

Angelina underwent a preliminary procedure called a nipple delay two weeks prior to her mastectomies. Tissue underneath the nipple was tested and came back as completely normal—no cancer or pre-cancer was found. This allowed Dr. Funk to leave the nipples and areolas intact. At the time of the mastectomy surgery, Angelina had a tissue expander put in place, along with allographic tissue.[11] The tissue expanders were gradually increased in size, and ten weeks after the mastectomies, the breast implants replaced the tissue expanders.

———————————— **MY JOURNEY** ————————————

I hadn't seen an old college friend in quite some time, and she seemed a bit dazzled that my breasts looked so "healthy," as she put it, especially considering our advancing ages. "Are they real?" she said, seeming to tease. "I'm just kidding. They look great."

I shook my head. "No, you're right. They're absolutely not," I said. "They're brand-new. The old ones tried to kill me."

Selena (Oklahoma City, Oklahoma)

Breast Implants and Saline Versus Silicone

Two types of implants can be inserted underneath the skin and chest muscle that remain after a mastectomy. This is usually done as part of a two- or three-stage procedure.

———————

11. Allograph: is a piece of cadaver skin that has had all the cells taken out of it, leaving the collagen. It is like a scaffold, which allows a patient's own cells and blood vessels to grow into it.

1. Stage one: The surgeon places a device called an expander under the chest muscle. The expander is slowly filled with saline during visits to the doctor after surgery.

2. Stage two: After the chest tissue has relaxed and healed sufficiently, the expander is removed and an implant is put in its place. The chest tissue is usually ready for the implant six weeks to six months after a mastectomy. Expanders can be put in place as part of either an immediate or a delayed reconstruction.

3. Stage three (optional): This involves re-creating a nipple-areola complex (NAC) on the reconstructed breast, which is discussed later in this chapter.

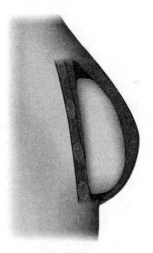

Breast Reconstruction with Implant
Source: © Alila Medical Media—*www.AlilaMedicalMedia.com*

Before making a decision about what's right for you, consider the following issues related to surgery and recovery:

- Will you have enough skin and muscle after a mastectomy to cover the implant?

- Implants usually mean a shorter operation, less blood loss, and a quicker recovery time than reconstruction with a flap.
- Multiple follow-up visits are needed to inflate the expander, and a second operation is required to insert the implant.

Possible complications include:

- Extrusion of the implant (the implant breaks through the skin)
- Implant rupture (saline or silicone leaks into surrounding tissue)
- Formation of hard scar tissue around the implant (known as a contracture)

You'll also need to consider that an implant may not last a lifetime. The longer you have one the more likely you'll be to develop complications and need to remove or replace the implant. Also, silicone implants may provide a more natural-looking breast shape than saline implants.

Table 1 clarifies some of the other differences.

Characteristic	Saline Implant	Silicone Implant
Components	Silicone shell filled with saltwater	Silicone shell with silicone gel interior
Texture	Not as soft as silicone	Soft, like natural breast tissue
Incision required	Shorter: implant is deflated when inserted	Longer: implant is full when inserted
Interior substance	Filled by surgeon during operation	Prefilled by manufacturer
Rupture	Obvious	May be undetected
Follow-up recommended	None	Periodic MRI screening

Table 1. *Source: Kathy Steligo, The Breast Reconstruction Guidebook: Issues and Answers from Research to Recovery* (Baltimore: Johns Hopkins, 2012).

Autologous Tissue Reconstruction:
What's All the Flap About?

This technique involves taking a piece of tissue containing skin, fat, blood vessels, and sometimes muscle from another place in a woman's body so it can be used to rebuild the breast. This piece of tissue is called a flap. Different locations in the body, such as fleshy areas, can provide flaps for breast reconstruction. They include three types of flaps:

1. *TRAM flap:* Tissue, including muscle, which comes from the lower abdomen. This is the most common type used in breast reconstruction.
2. *DIEP flap:* Tissue that comes from the abdomen, as in a TRAM flap, but contains only skin and fat.
3. *Latissimus dorsi flap:* Tissue that comes from the middle and side of the back.

Wherever the flaps come from, they can be either pedicled or free. With a pedicled flap, the tissue and attached blood vessels are moved together through the body to the breast area. With a free flap, the tissue is cut free from its blood supply and attached to new blood vessels in the breast area.

Tissue reconstruction may provide a more natural breast shape than implants and is less likely to be damaged by radiation therapy than implants.

Things to consider regarding surgery and recovery include these things:

- Longer surgical procedure than for implants; more blood loss
- Recovery period may be longer
- Pedicled flap reconstruction is a shorter operation than free flap but requires more donor tissue
- Free flap reconstruction uses less donor tissue than pedicled flap reconstruction but is a longer, highly technical operation

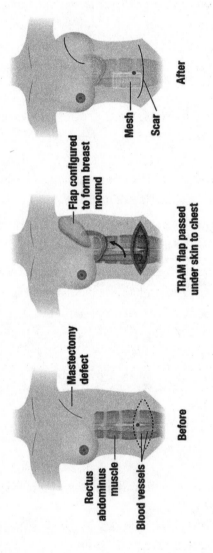

Reconstruction with Flap: Transverse Rectus Abdominis Myocutaneous (TRAM) Flap Surgery

Source: © Alila Medical Media—www.AlilaMedicalMedia.com

requiring a specialized surgeon with experience reattaching blood vessels

Possible complications include:

- Death of the transferred tissue (Necrosis)
- Blood clots
- Pain and weakness at the site from which the donor tissue was taken
- Obesity, diabetes, and smoking may increase the rate of complications
- Leaves a scar at the site from which the donor tissue was taken

―――――――――――― MY JOURNEY ――――――――――――

I'm in breast limbo right now. After losing one in a mastectomy, the other is just hanging around without a bra. My doctor tells me I should wait on a mastectomy bra until I finish chemo. So what's a girl to do? This is putting a crimp in my style, especially when I go out—even to the store!

I need to end up with two really natural-looking breasts. I know I've got enough tummy tissue for the TRAM flap procedure. I could do double D if that's the criteria! But I've heard some bad stuff about that, too, like how hard recovery can be and insurance companies don't always cover all of it, so I don't know what to do.

Until I figure it out, I'll keep dreaming of the perfect breast job that will keep me cancer-free and looking *good!*

Ayesha (Detroit, Michigan)

Suzanne Somers Used Belly Fat Stem Cells to Achieve Her Goals

Actress and ThighMaster guru Suzanne Somers was diagnosed with stage I breast cancer in 2001. She had a lumpectomy and radiation but declined chemotherapy. In 2012, she announced that she had undergone an experimental procedure to reconstruct her breast using her own fat cells.

Cosmetic and reconstructive surgeons have used this technique, called fat grafting, for decades. But Ms. Somers's surgeon, Dr. Joel Aronowitz, used a cutting edge, twenty-first-century version of the technique called adipose-derived stem cell (ADSC) transplantation. This procedure was so new at the time that Suzanne Somers was actually the first "human subject" in the United States enrolled in a research trial of ADSC transplantation.

According to Dr. Aronowitz, "Stem cell treatment has the advantage of producing a natural regrowth of fat tissue within the breast, giving it a soft, natural appearance and feel using the woman's own fat."

Adipose tissue is just another name for *fat*. However, fat tissue is made up of more than fat cells. It also contains stem cells, which are otherwise nondescript body cells with one incredibly important distinction. Since stem cells have the potential to grow and give rise to a variety of specialized tissues, these cells are one of the mainstays of the new field of regenerative medicine.

ADSC isolated from fat by liposuction have the remarkable property of being able to grow into a variety of tissues, including fat, muscle, cartilage, and blood vessels.

During the operation to reconstruct or improve the appearance of the breast, about two cups of fat are harvested from the belly, hips, and/or thighs using routine liposuction techniques. The fat is divided into two portions. One portion goes into a special machine, called a Celution®, that separates the fat from the stem cells. What comes out is a highly enriched mixture of ADSC. The mixture is combined with the other portion of unenriched fat and injected into the breast to fill in the defects. Although immediate results are seen, some loss of volume will occur, but the appearance slowly improves as the stem cells cause new fat tissue to grow.

According to Dr. Aronowitz, health insurance companies haven't yet decided to reimburse doctors for the ADSC transplant procedure, which adds about $2,500 to the surgery bill that many patients are willing to pay out of pocket. For those who can't afford this, they may be eligible to enroll in a clinical research trial that will pay for the procedure.

Check out Dr. Aronowitz's work at *http://www.breastpreservation foundation.org.*

Getting the NAC of It: Nipple Restoration and Medical Tattoos

Studies show that re-creating the nipple and areola, known as the nipple-areolar complex (NAC), has both psychological and aesthetic significance for many patients and symbolizes the transition from patient to survivor.

Nipple delay is a surgical procedure done in preparation for a nipple-sparing mastectomy (Chapter 4). The NAC must have its own supply of blood in order to remain healthy. If circulation to these tissues after a nipple-sparing mastectomy is inadequate, these structures can die and the dead tissue will have to be surgically removed.

A nipple-delay procedure is performed to create new blood vessel connections from the breast skin to the NAC in the hope that the nipples and areolas remain alive and well. It involves cutting the blood vessels and other breast tissue beneath the nipple so that it's no longer dependent on the tissue underneath it for its blood supply. The NAC then becomes accustomed to receiving its blood supply from the surrounding skin instead of from the breast tissue that lies underneath. This is a fairly uncommon procedure and is usually reserved for patients who have had breast surgery in the past.

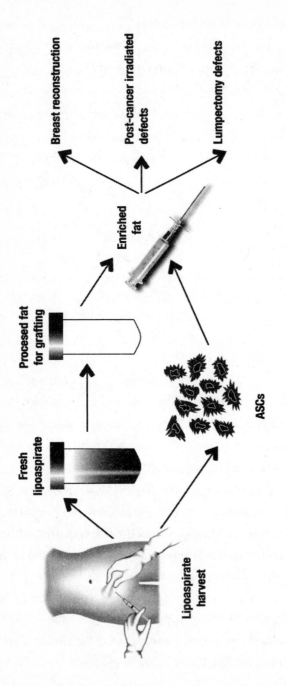

Fat Stem Cell Transplant

MY JOURNEY

It was so exciting to finally finish the journey of reconstruction. I had my breasts and nipples and areola done and soon my tattooing will be complete. It's been a long haul but I am so glad I decided to get nipples. The skin graft was painful, and I don't recommend doing it during the hottest part of the summer, but it was worth it. I mean, I look in the mirror now and I feel whole again, if such a thing is possible. My breasts will never be "natural" again, but I think they are beautiful in a brand-new way!

Kerry (Baltimore, Maryland)

After a non-nipple-sparing mastectomy and any necessary adjuvant therapy is completed, a woman has two choices for NAC restoration. A surgeon may reconstruct a new nipple by cutting and moving small pieces of skin from the reconstructed breast to the nipple site and sculpting them into a nipple shape. A few months after nipple reconstruction, the surgeon can re-create the areola, which is usually done using tattoo ink. However, in some cases, skin grafts may be taken from the groin or abdomen and attached to the breast to create an areola.

Another choice is to have a medical tattoo artist create a tattoo of the NAC, using special techniques to create a three-dimensional effect, which uses a broad range of color and adds shadows to give the nipple a raised, three-dimensional appearance. Tattoos can also include more realistic-looking areola, including details such as the tiny Montgomery glands surrounding the nipple.

Vinnie Myers and Stephanie Holvick, RN: Nipple Tattoo Artists

Once a renowned tattoo artist, Vinnie Myers has become a legend in breast cancer circles for his NAC tattoos. About five years ago,

Myers had become so busy doing nipple tattoos that he thought he might stop doing them. But fate intervened.

"The day I decided to stop is the day my sister called me and told me she had breast cancer," Meyers said. "I decided this is a sign that I've got to keep doing this."

Now, nipple tattooing is the only thing he does and he's had roughly 8,000 cancer survivors come through his door.

In October 2015, Myers told the *Today* show, "When you're looking at those breasts, all you see are the scars, and all you're reminded of is cancer. So when you put this finishing touch on there, it distracts your eye from all those other imperfections because you have something to look at that's very pleasing, and it's an incredibly emotional finishing touch."

In 2015, Myers was featured in an episode of *Botched*, an E! network show about two Los Angeles surgeons, Doctors Paul Nassif and Terry Dubrow, who specialize in fixing plastic surgery mistakes or complications.

NAC tattoos are a billable medical procedure and cost approximately $250 to $400 per breast. Most health insurance should cover the procedure, as the Women's Health and Breast Cancer Right Act of 1990 requires coverage for all aspects of breast reconstruction. Many medical tattoo artists offer free services for those who are unable to pay out of pocket or are not covered by insurance.

For women interested in having nipple tattooing, Stephanie Holvick, RN, a nurse turned medical tattooist, says it's important that they do their homework. This can include getting a recommendation or referral from their surgeon, meeting with a practitioner prior to the procedure to discuss their experience, and viewing their previous work to make sure that they feel comfortable in the setting.

Some women may feel more comfortable in a medical office than a tattoo parlor, but according to Holvick, tattoo body artists generally do excellent work and it's good that clients have choices.

According to Ms. Holvick, "NAC tattooing is about empowerment. It's nice to help these women feel put back together."

One of her patients, Maria Wylan, said, "Whenever I look at myself in the mirror, I don't feel scarred. It looks beautiful."

─────────────── MY JOURNEY ───────────────

Once a woman feels together enough to stop looking backward and be in the moment, she is ready to accept her new body and make peace with it. No matter how long it's been since surgery and whatever other treatment you may have had, the hardest thing to do is come to terms with the fact that your body will never look—or feel—the same again. In fact, for some of you, it may actually improve! "New and Improved," like some favorite product at the store, right?

As far as nipple reconstruction, I had no idea what they would look like, especially since I could hardly comprehend that my originals were gone, replaced by some newfangled version of whatever it is we use to identify ourselves as women. That's loaded enough, without the nipple question. But, anyway, I went ahead, hoping my new nipples would help me feel more feminine and complete. I wanted to get my husband excited again, but I wasn't sure how I could do that, even though he's been great and not freaked out at all about my changed body. Regardless, I needed those nipples for me, first, and I am so glad I moved forward on this journey.

Dalia (Atlanta, Georgia)

A Personal Choice

For any woman with breast cancer, contemplating breast reconstruction is a very personal matter and often presents real turmoil in choosing what feels right.

Dr. Marisa Weiss is chief medical officer of *Breastcancer.org*. She has found that while prioritizing their goals for reconstruction, most of her patients tend to rank receiving the most effective anticancer therapy above and beyond anything else, including reconstruction. Then they tend to favor whatever will sustain their ability to function fully and comfortably after recovering from the reconstruction procedure. As far as aesthetics are concerned, Weiss reports that her patients are looking first at how the reconstructed breast feels and looks as far as size, shape, and symmetry with the other breast. And, of course, there are the usual practical considerations like timing, cost, availability, and length of recovery.

Once you get the proper advice and counsel from the appropriate medical professionals, breast reconstruction comes down to a woman—and her partner if there is one—making a very personal choice.

As Dr. Aronowitz and his famous patient Suzanne Somers advise: "Don't get locked in or talked into the first thing your doctor may recommend. Do your own research. Ask a lot of questions. Decide for yourself."

──────────── **MY JOURNEY** ────────────

Here's my advice to the ladies: When it comes to your husband, make it crystal clear what you need and want from him. Start by reminding him that you are still a woman—a complete (sort of) healthy one, too—from head to toe. Have him touch you to prove it! You're supposed to be in this together, so even if you feel like you're alone on an island, you're not, and your man probably wants you to help him through the struggle as much as he's helping you. Fear, be gone! There's no time for that, not when it comes to owning—and loving—who you are.

Joan (Charlotte, North Carolina)

KEY POINTS TO REMEMBER

✓ Oncoplastic surgery has two goals: to effectively treat cancer and to restore a natural shape and appearance to the breast.

✓ Breasts can be rebuilt with saline or silicone implants, or with a patient's own body tissues using flaps.

✓ Fat grafting uses liposuction fat from a patient's belly or thighs to fill in tissue defects following cancer surgery and to repair damage caused by radiation treatments.

✓ For many patients, re-creation of the nipple and areola symbolizes the transition from patient to survivor.

✓ Breast reconstruction and nipple tattoos are a billable medical procedure and should be covered by your health insurance.

✓ Take your time and do your research in deciding what's right for you.

GONE!

When it first fell out, I knew it was time to let it rain.
Why pretend?

On a lovely Saturday afternoon I sent my boys away,
to leave Mommy alone to her own devices.

My surgical tools removed it all Godspeed,
a scalp in hand as if I'd slain the beast.

My youngest boy came home and told me I looked weird.
The middle one couldn't resist elaborating.

"Uh, Mom, it's weird, but kinda cool."
Luckily, my biggest boy still loved his wife.

And now, my body has been turned into a construction site
with two less breasts and who knows yet what else.

My hair has grown back just in time to give shade to tattoos.
Luckily, my biggest boy still loves his wife.

And my sons don't know how cool I've really become.

—Anonymous

6 OVARIAN CANCER: Rewriting the Textbooks

Cancer changes your life, often for the better.
You learn what's important, you learn to prioritize,
and you learn not to waste your time.
You tell people you love them.
My friend Gilda Radner (who died of ovarian cancer
in 1989 at age forty-two) used to say,
"If it wasn't for the downside,
having cancer would be the best thing and
everyone would want it."
That's true.
If it wasn't for the downside.

—Joel Siegel, *Good Morning America*

A Stunning Paradigm Shift

The new name for so-called ovarian cancer is pelvic serous carcinoma (PSC). And it's not a cancer of the ovaries at all. This cancer arises in the finger-like projections (fimbriae) at the ends of the fallopian tubes.

This rather shocking discovery came about as a result of patients like Angelina Jolie, women who are carriers of BRCA1 and BRCA2 mutations who have had their ovaries and fallopian tubes removed to prevent cancer from developing (Chapter 3). When pathologists studied these ovaries and tubes, they found precancerous changes or early cancer in up to 17 percent of cases. But these discoveries were always seen in the fallopian tubes, never the ovaries. These findings were then extended to include nonhereditary ovarian cancers as well.

Because this cancer has been traditionally considered one of the most common gynecologic cancers and the fifth most frequent cause of cancer death in women (per the NCI), this new model—defining what we previously referred to as ovarian cancer as pelvic serous carcinoma—may have huge implications for future treatment and prevention of the disease.

The potential impact for patients could be immense. If what we have called ovarian cancer actually comes from the fallopian tubes, surgeons in the future might have to remove only the tubes and not the ovaries of patients like Angelina Jolie, thus sparing them forced menopause, infertility, and other medical problems.

Studies are underway to assess whether a salpingectomy (removal of the fallopian tubes) alone will be as protective as removing the tubes *and* ovaries, and which patients would be the best candidates for the less drastic surgery.

Basic Anatomy and Function

The ovaries and fallopian tubes are a pair of organs in the female reproductive system, located in the pelvis, one on each side of the uterus. The ovaries make eggs and the female hormones, estrogen and progesterone. The fallopian tubes are a pair of long, slender tunnels through which eggs pass on their way from the ovaries to the uterus.

The uterus, ovaries, and fallopian tubes all exist in what's called the peritoneal cavity, which separates the abdominal and pelvic organs from the inner wall of the abdomen.

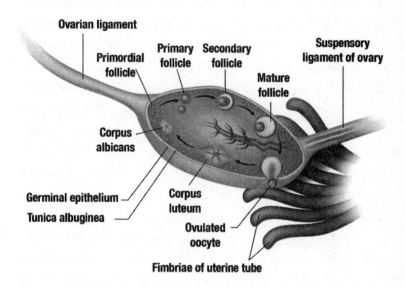

The Anatomy of the Ovary and Fallopian Tube
Source: Alila Medical Media (*Shutterstock.com*)

Ovarian (Pelvic Serous) Cancer:
The Fundamental Facts

Ovarian cancer (PSC) accounts for approximately 3 percent of all cancers among women in the United States. Latest figures from 2014 report an estimated 22,000 women diagnosed with PSC in the United States, and approximately 14,000 will eventually die of the disease.

The good news is that the incidence of PSC has decreased by 1 percent each year between 1987 and 2011, and the mortality rates fell an average of 1.6 percent a year between 2001 and 2010.

PSC has the highest mortality of all cancers of the female reproductive system. This reflects, in part, a lack of early symptoms and effective cancer screening tests. As a result, PSC is often diagnosed at an advanced stage after the cancer has spread beyond the ovary. White women have higher incidence and mortality rates than women of other racial and ethnic groups.

MY JOURNEY

For several months I wasn't feeling well, but I didn't think I had cancer until I came across a list of ovarian cancer symptoms online and realized I had them all! Something clicked. I knew I had cancer right then and there, so I called my doctor and told him my gut impulse said cancer. It turned out I was right. Thank God I listened to myself and followed my instincts, in spite of all the noise on the Internet, because we caught it early enough that my prognosis is quite good.

Britt (Salem, Oregon)

What Are the Risk Factors?

Anything that increases the chances of an individual getting a disease can be considered a risk factor. They include the following:

- *Family history of cancer:* Women who have a close female relative on either side of the family with PSC have an increased risk of the disease. Women of Jewish ancestry and/or with a family history of cancers of the breast, uterus, pancreas, colon or rectum, or male breast cancer, may also have an increased risk of PSC.

- *Personal history of breast cancer:* Women who have had cancer of the breast, uterus, colon, or rectum have a higher risk of PSC.
- *Age over fifty-five:* Most women are over age fifty-five when diagnosed.
- *Never pregnant:* Older women who have never been pregnant.
- *Menopausal hormone therapy:* Some studies have suggested that women who take estrogen by itself (without progesterone) for ten-plus years may have an increased risk.

The Role of Genes in Pelvic Serous Cancer

PSC can be caused by gene mutations that are inherited from parents. These hereditary cases of PSC make up approximately 5 to 10 percent of all cases. Many of these are due to the hereditary breast and ovarian cancer genes, BRCA1 and BRCA2, described in Chapter 3. However, other genes, including those that cause Lynch Syndrome (Chapter 7), can also be involved in this disease.

Regardless of whether PSC is hereditary or nonhereditary (sporadic), mutation of a gene called TP53 seems to be an early event in the development of these cancers. The normal function of TP53 is to be the "guardian of our genomes" by helping our cells repair environmental damage to our DNA and also helping cells "commit suicide" if the DNA damage is too severe. If damage to the TP53 itself occurs, loss of its guardian function leads to genetic instability and more mutations that eventually cause cancer.

Family History = Increased Risk

Women with one first-degree relative (mother, daughter, or sister) with a history of PSC have an increased risk of being diagnosed with PSC. This risk is higher in women who have one first-degree relative and one second-degree relative (grandmother or aunt) with a history of PSC. This risk is even higher in women who have two or more first-degree relatives with a history of PSC.

Cassandra and Charlotte Brosnan: Losing a Wife and Daughter

Actor Pierce Brosnan knows the devastation PSC can cause. In 1991, the former star of multiple *James Bond* films lost his wife, actress Cassandra Harris, to the disease. And in 2013, their daughter, Charlotte Brosnan, lost her three-year battle with the same disease.

Unfortunately, the Brosnan family knew this day could come. Not only did Charlotte's mother die of PSC but also her grandmother died of it. This family medical history (shown here as a pedigree diagram) strongly suggests an inherited genetic cause for the disease. In fact, Charlotte had been receiving regular checkups to detect PSC. (For more information on pedigree diagrams and how genetic counselors use them to diagnose cancers that run in families, see Chapter 3.)

Some women with an increased risk of ovarian cancer may choose to have a prophylactic salpingo-oophorectomy, which involves the removal of healthy fallopian tubes and ovaries so that cancer cannot grow in them. In high-risk women, this procedure has been shown to greatly decrease the risk of developing PSC.

Angelina Jolie-Pitt: The Safe Side

As described in Chapter 3, actress Angelina Jolie-Pitt underwent prophylactic bilateral mastectomies in 2013, based on her family medical history and testing positive for mutations in the BRCA1 gene.

For two years after her mastectomies, doctors followed Angelina very closely for any early signs of PSC. This screening included blood tests looking for a PSC-associated biomarker called CA-125, as well as other less specific biomarkers of inflammation.

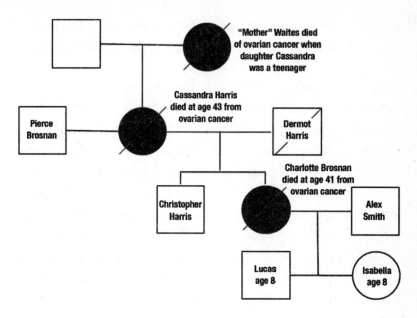

Pedigree of Charlotte Brosnon
Source: *CelebrityDiagnosis.com*

In March 2015, when her blood work showed some early signs of inflammation, Jolie-Pitt underwent an ultrasound, a CT scan, and a PET scan. Fortunately, no tumors were found, although the possibility of a very early stage cancer could not be completely ruled out. After speaking to many doctors, surgeons, and naturopaths, Ms. Jolie-Pitt decided to undergo a laparoscopic bilateral salpingo-oophorectomy. In other words, she had both her ovaries and fallopian tubes removed. No signs of cancer were found.

> **NOTE to PATIENT:**
> A majority of women (90 to 95 percent) with nonhereditary pelvic serous cancer (PSC) do not have a hereditary basis for their disease.

Evelyn Lauder:
Wife, Businesswoman, Survivor, and Advocate

As a child, Evelyn and her family fled Nazi-occupied Austria and came to live in New York City. There she met her future husband, Leonard, son of Estée Lauder. After their marriage, she became active in a then fledgling cosmetics company, naming the Clinique line and becoming the head of Fragrance Development worldwide.

Evelyn Lauder was diagnosed with breast cancer in 1989. That same year, she spearheaded a fund-raising drive that brought in $18 million to establish the Evelyn H. Lauder Breast Center at Memorial Sloan-Kettering Cancer Center in New York City. Shortly after its opening in 1992, it became the nation's first comprehensive breast cancer center, incorporating diagnostic and treatment services under one roof.

Shortly after, she and friend Alexandra Penney, the editor of *Self* magazine, created the pink ribbon, which has become the worldwide symbol of breast health. And in 1993, she founded the Breast Cancer Research Foundation, a nonprofit organization that has since raised more than $350 million to fight the disease.

Ms. Lauder was diagnosed with nongenetic ovarian cancer in 2007. She died at home with her family in New York City in November 2011.

The following statement is on the BCRF website:

> The Breast Cancer Research Foundation mourns the loss of our visionary Founder and Chairman, Evelyn Lauder. Her passionate action and determination to improve the health of women and their families led her to establish BCRF. Her single-minded dedication to finding a cure for breast cancer never wavered.

What Are the Symptoms?

Early ovarian cancer may not cause obvious symptoms. But, as the cancer grows, symptoms may include any or all of the following:

- Pain, swelling, or a feeling of pressure in the abdomen or pelvis
- Vaginal bleeding that is heavy or irregular, especially after menopause
- Vaginal discharge that is clear, white, or colored with blood
- A lump in the pelvic area
- Gastrointestinal problems, such as gas, bloating, or constipation
- Feeling very tired all the time

--------------------------- MY JOURNEY ---------------------------

Since there is no test or screening for ovarian cancer, as with other cancers, like the smear test for cervical cancer, women have to be extra vigilant about paying attention to any symptoms they may have. Not that we should be paranoid about every ache or itch, because most women have plenty of those. But still, everybody should be aware that early diagnosis is the key to a good outcome. I mean, your survival may depend on it! So if you have symptoms—any kind of unusual stuff—don't take any chances! Even if you're not sure, check with your doctor. What are they going to do, get mad at you and cut you off as a patient? Thank God I didn't wait when I started feeling odd. Ovarian cancer can show up real quick and kill you even quicker.

Evelyn (Denver, Colorado)

Kathy Bates: "Doing What I Love to Do"

Academy Award–winning actress Kathy Bates was diagnosed with ovarian cancer in 2003. While traveling in Europe, she felt bloated and threw up a few times. Although she originally chalked it up to the travel, she listened to her body, which was telling her that something was wrong. She went to her gynecologist as soon as she got home and an ultrasound test revealed a mass in her right ovary. Her treatment included surgery and chemotherapy.

Bates also had a strong history of breast cancer in her family but tested negative for genetic mutations associated with the disease. But in July 2012, Bates announced that she had recently undergone bilateral mastectomies for breast cancer. She did not require radiation or chemotherapy, and doctors gave her a good prognosis.

"My doctors have assured me I'm going to be around for a long time," she told *People* magazine. "I'm looking forward to getting back to work doing what I love to do."

Diagnosing Pelvic Serous Cancer

Any initial evaluation of a patient suspected of having cancer begins with a thorough patient history and general physical examination. If the genitourinary system is under suspicion, a pelvic exam will also be performed.

A pelvic exam is made up of two parts. First, a speculum is inserted into the vagina and the doctor or nurse looks at the vagina and cervix for signs of disease. A Pap test, which uses a special brush to remove some of the cells of the cervix, is typically done at this time, too. The brush is sent to the laboratory where the cells will be examined for any signs of cancer.

The second part of the pelvic exam is called the bimanual exam.

The doctor or nurse inserts one or two lubricated, gloved fingers of one hand into the vagina and places the other hand over the lower abdomen. He or she is able to feel the size, shape, and position of the uterus and ovaries between their two hands.

Imaging Studies and Laboratory Tests

A variety of techniques may be used to "see" the cancer inside the body, in this case to specifically aid in diagnosing ovarian cancer. These methods include the following:

- *Ultrasound exam:* A procedure in which high-energy sound waves (ultrasound) are bounced off internal tissues or organs in the abdomen and make echoes. The echoes form a picture of body tissues called a sonogram.
- *Transvaginal ultrasound:* An ultrasound probe connected to a computer is inserted into the patient's vagina and gently moved to show different organs.
- *CT scan* (CAT scan): Converts a series of X-ray pictures taken at different angles into a three-dimensional image of the part of the body being examined.
- *MRI* (magnetic resonance imaging): Uses a magnet, radio waves, and a computer to make a series of detailed pictures of areas inside the body.
- *PET scan* (positron emission tomography scan): A small amount of radioactive glucose (sugar) is injected into a vein. The PET scanner rotates around the body, making a picture of where glucose is being used in the body. Malignant tumor cells show up brighter in the picture because they are more active and take up more glucose than normal cells do.
- *CA-125 assay:* A test that measures the level of CA-125 in the blood. CA-125 is a substance released by cells into the

bloodstream. An increased CA-125 level can be a sign of cancer or another condition, such as endometriosis.

- *Biopsy:* Once a tumor is located, a portion of it is removed and sent to the lab to be examined under a microscope by a pathologist, who will determine the type of tumor, whether it is malignant (cancerous) or benign, and the grade of the tumor (see Grading Tumors Chapter 1).

After cancer has been diagnosed, additional tests determine if cancer cells have spread within the ovaries or to other parts of the body. This allows the cancer to be assigned a stage (Chapter 1), which has implications for treatment and prognosis.

The prognosis (chance of recovery) and treatment options depend on the following:

- The stage and grade of the cancer
- The type and size of the tumor
- Whether all of the tumor can be removed by surgery
- Any swelling of the abdomen
- The patient's age and general health
- If the cancer has just been diagnosed or has recurred (come back)

─────────────── **MY JOURNEY** ───────────────

I started having periods at sixteen, and they were always irregular and often included terrible pain in my legs and hips. I even threw up and felt like my stomach would explode at any minute. My first pap smear revealed multiple cysts on my ovaries, which were never biopsied. The doctors put me through a battery of tests, but no one could explain anything. This went on for several years, until I couldn't keep seeing a doctor because I lost my health insurance. Finally, when

I *could* manage to see a doctor, he did a biopsy, which revealed that a carcinoma around my ovary had spread to my liver. The surgeon wasn't sure it was ovarian cancer, but, to be safe, he removed just about everything: both ovaries, my uterus, a foot of my bowel, the stomach lining, my appendix, spleen, and a piece of my liver. I had just turned twenty-five.

Since then, my condition has gone up and down, and while I keep hoping for the best, not a day goes by when I wonder why I wasn't more assertive about my health when I was younger, and why I just accepted the verdict of my regular doctor. If I've learned anything from this, it's that each of us has to look out for ourselves because no one else will go to the mat for you unless you demand it.

Kadesha (Milwaukee, Wisconsin)

Treatments

Most patients with the symptoms previously mentioned will undergo surgery to remove as much tumor as possible. This is called cytoreductive surgery or tumor debulking, and its aim is to reduce the amount of cancer before beginning chemotherapy.

Patients may then take chemotherapy drugs, such as cisplatin and paclitaxel, injected directly into the peritoneal cavity where any residual cancer cells may reside following the tumor debulking procedure. They also receive systemic chemotherapy with drugs, such as taxane and platinum, which are injected into their veins to kill any cancer cells that have metastasized to other parts of the body.

For PSCs that become resistant to platinum therapy, bevacizumab (Avastin) is an FDA approved treatment for these patients. This is a drug that "starves" tumors of their blood supplies. A drug called olaparib (Lynparza) is FDA approved to treat advanced PSCs in patients with BRCA1 and BRCA2 mutations, but only after traditional chemotherapies have been tried.

Hormonal Side Effects of Treatment

Women who have had both ovaries removed will no longer be able to become pregnant. The loss of both ovaries also eliminates the body's source of sex hormones, causing premature menopause. Soon after surgery, menopausal symptoms are likely, including hot flashes and vaginal dryness. If they prove troublesome, hormone replacement therapy (HRT) may be in order.

As previously discussed, actress Angelina Jolie-Pitt underwent prophylactic removal of both of her ovaries because she was considered at high risk for ovarian cancer. In her op-ed piece in the *New York Times*,[12] Angelina stated that she had been planning for this for some time and knew that she would be going into menopause. "I was readying myself physically and emotionally, discussing options with doctors, researching alternative medicine, and mapping my hormones for estrogen or progesterone replacement."

As a result of her research, she came to a momentous decision. "I have a little clear patch that contains bio-identical estrogen. A progesterone IUD was inserted in my uterus. It will help me maintain a hormonal balance, but, more important, it will help prevent uterine cancer. I chose to keep my uterus because cancer in that location is not part of my family history.'"

Looking Forward to the Future

Research is being done to test whether a tubectomy or salpingectomy (removal of only the fallopian tube) might be as effective as an

---

12. *http://www.nytimes.com/2015/03/24/opinion/angelina-jolie-pitt-diary-of-a-surgery.html?_r=0*

oophorectomy (removal of the ovary) for the prophylactic treatment of women at high risk of ovarian cancer. This would allow a woman to still have a menstrual cycle while eliminating forced menopause. A couple could still have a biologic child through in vitro fertilization and completing the pregnancy in a surrogate mother.

Tubectomy alone would also prevent additional problems that premenopausal women who lose their ovaries may suffer. These include increased risks of cardiovascular disease, Parkinsonism, cognitive impairment, depression, and anxiety.

Every year, thousands of women undergo hysterectomies for noncancerous conditions, tubal ligations, and other pelvic surgeries. If doctors also removed the fallopian tubes during these procedures, it could prove to substantially reduce the chances of these women developing so-called ovarian cancer. More research will give us the answer to this important question.

KEY POINTS TO REMEMBER

✓ What medical experts have traditionally called ovarian cancer probably arises in the fallopian tubes, and this could have a big impact on diagnosis and treatment in the future.

✓ The new name for ovarian cancer is pelvic serous carcinoma (PSC).

✓ PSC accounts for approximately 3 percent of all cancers in women and is the fifth leading cause of cancer-related death among women in the United States.

✓ PSC has the highest mortality of all cancers of the female reproductive system.

✓ Some PSCs are caused by inherited gene mutations, the most common being BRCA1 and BRCA2 and Lynch Syndrome.

✓ Women with one first-degree relative (mother, daughter, or sister) who have had PSC or have a family history of breast, uterine, colon, or pancreatic cancers, have an increased risk of developing PSC.

✓ Early PSC may not cause obvious symptoms.

✓ There are two new drugs (Avastin and Lynparza) to treat PSC in some women if traditional chemotherapy treatments stop working.

✓ Jewish women are at an increased risk for PSC.

✓ All women with PSC are candidates for genetic counseling and testing.

FRIED GRAY MATTER

It has now been proven
Chemo Brain is real.
As if we didn't notice
memory has turned
into a dog off leash
in a park full of hotdog buns.
Some days, mind is puppeting
feet and keys well as a Bud ad,
on other days my nose
is close to the green stew
of choice and darting
from should to could
to reruns I can follow
nearly as well as faking.

—Claudia Carlson

7

FROM IGNORANCE TO TENACITY: Learning About Uterine and Endometrial Cancers

I liked her so much. I couldn't get enough of her.

—Mel Brooks, speaking to SiriusXM
about his late wife, Anne Bancroft,
who died from uterine cancer in 2005

A Few Facts

According to the National Comprehensive Cancer Network, a nonprofit alliance of twenty-six cancer centers throughout the United States, cancer of the endometrium—also known as endometrial cancer, or simply uterine cancer—is the most common malignancy of the female reproductive system found among American women. The average chance of a woman being diagnosed with uterine cancer during her lifetime is about one in thirty-seven. Rates of this cancer are slightly higher among white women than African American women, but, unfortunately, black women are more likely to die from the disease.

The overall five-year survival rate, which reflects the percentage of people who survive at least five years after the cancer is first diagnosed, is 82 percent. It jumps to 95 percent if the cancer has not spread beyond the uterus at the time of diagnosis. Because most women with uterine cancer have early symptoms (abnormal vaginal bleeding, most commonly after menopause), about 75 percent of patients have cancer that has not spread beyond the uterus at the time of diagnosis.

About 5 percent of women who develop uterine cancer do so because of inherited mutations in their DNA and usually develop this disease ten or twenty years earlier than other patients who develop uterine cancer. Women with these inherited DNA mutations are said to have Lynch syndrome, which increases their risk of developing cancer in the colon and other organs, as well.

As is the case with several other cancers, our understanding of uterine cancer is being redefined by DNA studies that have already led to new ideas about better treatments.

Basic Anatomy and Function

The uterus is a hollow, muscular organ located in a woman's pelvis, which is where a fetus grows. In most nonpregnant women, the uterus is about three inches long. The lower, narrow end of the uterus is the cervix, which leads to the vagina.

The myometrium is the name for the layers of smooth muscle that make up the substance of the uterus. The endometrium, which covers the inner surface, is made up of glandular material and functions as a lining for the uterus.

The endometrium is made up of two layers. The basal layer lies

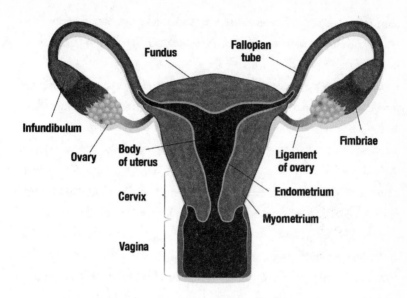

Anatomy of the Uterus: Female Reproductive System
Source: *istock.com*

next to the myometrium, beneath the functional layer. It is not shed at any time during the menstrual cycle. The functional layer develops from the basal layer.

The functional layer is the innermost surface of the uterus. This layer grows to a thick, blood vessel–rich, glandular tissue under the influence of the hormones estrogen—followed by progesterone—over the course of a menstrual cycle. It is adapted to provide an optimum environment for the implantation and growth of the embryo. During menstruation, this layer is completely shed.

Which Cancer Is It—Endometrium or Uterine?

Uterine cancer can start in different parts of the uterus. Most uterine cancers start in the endometrium, which forms the inner lining of the uterus. This is called endometrial cancer. Most endometrial cancers are considered to be adenocarcinomas—cancers that begin in cells that make mucus and other fluids.

Uterine sarcoma is an uncommon form of uterine cancer that forms in the muscle and tissue that support the uterus.

Risk Factors

Anything that increases one's risk of getting a disease is called a risk factor. Regarding endometrial cancer, risk factors include:

- Obesity, high blood pressure, or diabetes
- Family history of endometrial cancer in a first-degree relative (mother, sister, daughter)
- Family history of uterine, ovarian, or colon cancer, or Lynch syndrome (formerly known as hereditary nonpolyposis colon cancer or HNPCC)

What Is Lynch Syndrome?

Dr. Henry T. Lynch directs the Hereditary Cancer Center at Creighton University School of Medicine in Omaha, Nebraska. In the early 1960s, while still a medical student, Lynch began gathering evidence to show that some cancers have a genetic cause. The prevailing wisdom at the time surmised that cancer was a disease caused by environmental factors, not changes in DNA, and the National Institutes of Health repeatedly turned down funding for Lynch's work. But Dr. Lynch persisted, and his research laid one of the foundations for the way we understand cancer today.

His research, and therefore his findings, almost didn't happen for reasons other than a lack of grant funding. Before Henry Lynch entered medical school, he was a professional boxer under the stage name "Hammerin' Hank." Perhaps this first career instilled in him the dogged determination he needed to overcome early rejection of his work by the established experts.

The syndrome named after Henry Lynch is a hereditary cancer predisposition, which in affected patients and families creates high risks for developing a wide variety of cancers. The two most common tumors are cancers of the colon and uterus.

Lynch syndrome is caused by defects in the machinery that fixes DNA damage in our cells and involves four DNA mismatch repair (MMR) genes named MLH1, MSH2, MSH6, PMS2, and a fifth gene called EPCAM. When even one of these genes is abnormal, our DNA accumulates stutters, that is, short repetitions of the letters in our DNA code. These stutters are referred to as microsatellite instability (MSI).

Women affected by Lynch syndrome have a 10 to 53 percent chance of developing colon cancer by age seventy. They also have a 15 to 71 percent chance of developing uterine cancer by the same age.

> **NOTE to PATIENT:**
> If any type of cancer seems to run in your family,
> insist that your primary healthcare provider
> refer you to a certified genetic counselor.
> Or you can get in touch with one through the National
> Society of Genetic Counselors at *www.nsgc.org/*.

Patients affected by Lynch syndrome benefit from frequent, meticulous screening tests intensive designed to catch precancerous conditions before they develop into cancer. For more information, visit *http://www.ihavelynchsyndrome.com/*

Colonoscopy is recommended every one to two years beginning between the ages of twenty and twenty-five, or every two to five years before the youngest diagnosis of colon cancer in the family if diagnosed before the age of twenty-five. If the status of the patient's MMR genes is known, these intervals may be adjusted based on varying risks.

Starting between the ages of thirty and thirty-five, screening for uterine cancer should be done annually by pelvic examination and a sampling of endometrial tissues for assessment to look for precancerous changes.

The value of increased screening for other types of cancer is currently unknown. This topic should be discussed with your doctor and genetic counselor. For more information on hereditary cancers and the importance of genetic counseling, see Chapter 3.

Camille Grammar: Knowing Your Family History Can Save Your Life

As a cast member of *The Real Housewives of Beverly Hills*, Camille Grammar knew plenty about dealing with drama. But this knowledge didn't prepare her at all for the drama that entered her life in 2013.

Camille knew that cancer ran in her family: her grandmother had endometrial cancer when her mother was young, and her mother was diagnosed with stage III ovarian cancer when she was forty-seven years old. At the age of thirty-five, Camille decided to be tested for genetic markers and learned that she had Lynch syndrome. Her doctors strongly encouraged her to undergo a hysterectomy, but Camille was not yet ready to enter menopause and opted instead for close observation. Twice a year she had an endometrial biopsy, and in 2013 she received the devastating news that she had developed stage III endometrial cancer.

Camille underwent a radical hysterectomy at MD Anderson Cancer Center in Houston, Texas, and then received several rounds of chemotherapy and radiation therapy.

With her cancer now in remission, Camille is raising awareness about "below the belt" female cancers. Camille points out that these cancers can be silent killers because of the rampant lack of knowledge about the symptoms and the tendency for women to feel embarrassed to talk about diseases "below the belt," both of which increase the risk that the cancers will go undiagnosed until they have progressed to later—and much more dangerous—stages.

"I'm a survivor," Camille says, "and we're going to raise awareness to help other women in our position to survive and beat this."

> **NOTE to PATIENT:**
> Know your family history!

The Role of Estrogen

Your body makes the hormone estrogen, which helps develop and maintain your female sex characteristics. It regulates the growth and thickening of the endometrium as well as other aspects of the menstrual cycle. Because of these effects, estrogen can affect the growth of some cancers, including endometrial cancer.

Being exposed to estrogen increases a woman's risk of developing endometrial cancer, and it can happen several ways, as we describe here.

Estrogen-Only Hormone Replacement Therapy

Estrogen may be taken to replace the estrogen no longer produced by the ovaries in postmenopausal women or women whose ovaries have been removed. This is called hormone replacement therapy (HRT). The use of estrogen-only HRT increases the risk of endometrial hyperplasia, an abnormal thickening of the endometrium in postmenopausal women. Although it is not cancer, in some cases it may lead to endometrial cancer. Therefore, estrogen-only therapy is usually recommended only for women who do not have a uterus. When estrogen is combined with progestin (combination estrogen-progestin replacement therapy), the risk of endometrial cancer in postmenopausal women does not increase; however, the combination *does* increase the risk of breast cancer, heart disease, stroke, and blood clots.

Three factors affect estrogen in the body: 1) Early menstruation—beginning menstrual periods at an early age increases the number of years the body is exposed to estrogen; 2) late menopause—women who reach menopause at an older age are exposed to estrogen for a longer time; and 3) never being pregnant—because estrogen levels are lower during pregnancy, women who have never been pregnant are exposed to estrogen for a longer time than women who have been pregnant.

Tamoxifen

This is one of a group of drugs called selective estrogen receptor modulators, or SERMs (Chapter 2). Tamoxifen acts like estrogen on some tissues in the body, such as the uterus, but blocks the effects of estrogen on other tissues, such as the breast.

Tamoxifen is used to prevent breast cancer in women who are at high risk for the disease. However, using tamoxifen for more than two years increases the risk of endometrial cancer, a risk that is greater in postmenopausal women.

It is recommended that any patient taking this drug should have a pelvic exam every year and should report any vaginal bleeding (other than menstrual bleeding) as soon as possible.

--------------------- **MY JOURNEY** ---------------------

Getting diagnosed with endometrial uterine cancer at the age of thirty-four was no picnic. Thank God I already had two kids because once I lost most of what physically makes me a woman, I felt empty. It wasn't just the early onset of menopause. My whole psyche was messed up for a long time.

Raising my kids is the only thing that kept me sane, but using that word—*sane*—may be giving myself too much credit. At first, I was just damaged from the surgery and treatments, probably not much different from anyone else who has had so much of their insides removed. But soon enough, the whole cycle my body and mind had grown accustomed to since I was a teenager went missing! *Gone!* I didn't know how to behave. All the hot flashes, mood swings, and depression were so out of character for me, yet they were what dominated my days until I finally was able to come to grips with my changed body and the way I feel about it. And I'm still working on it.

Randy (Las Vegas, Nevada)

Symptoms of Endometrial Cancer

These and other signs and symptoms may be caused by endometrial cancer or other conditions. Check with your doctor if you have any of the following:

- Bleeding or discharge not related to menstruation (periods)
- Difficult or painful urination
- Pain during sexual intercourse
- Pain in the pelvic area

Fran Drescher and
the Importance of Tenacity

Nearly two decades ago, the actress best known for her role as nanny Fran Fine on the TV show *The Nanny* knew something was wrong with her. "For two years," Drescher says, "I was bleeding twenty-four/seven and being prescribed different treatments that did not work. It was easier to treat the problem if it was benign, and that's the kind of treatment I got, including doses of estrogen, which only make uterine cancer grow. Despite the fact that the doctors and I heard hooves galloping, we were looking for horses not zebras."

In 2000, after two years and eight different doctors, Fran finally got the correct diagnosis: stage I endometrial cancer. She underwent a radical hysterectomy and did not need any chemotherapy or radiation.

In a June 2014 interview with *lifechangingmoments.com*, Drescher said she doesn't blame the doctors for the delay in her diagnosis. "I blame myself as much as those doctors. We have become infantile because we let the doctors make our decisions for us. But I'm a bit of a control freak, and I kept going to doctors, so my pursuit of the right answers was my own growth from ignorance through tenacity. I realize no one else should have power of attorney over my body."

In 2002, Fran wrote a book, *Cancer Schmancer*, about her difficult journey from symptoms to diagnosis. During a book tour, she realized that many other women had gone through very similar experiences. She realized the book was "not the end, but rather the beginning of a life mission to improve women's healthcare in America."

Now cancer-free for over ten years, Drescher started the Cancer Schmancer Movement and Cancer Schmancer Foundation, with the goal of transforming women from patients into medical consumers, and to shift this nation's priority from searching for a cancer cure toward prevention and early detection.

Diagnosing and Treating Endometrial Cancer

Because endometrial cancer begins inside the uterus, it does not usually show up in the results of a Pap test. For this reason, a sample of endometrial tissue must be removed and checked under a microscope to look for cancer cells. Several procedures may be used.

Endometrial Biopsy

The procedure removes tissue from the endometrium (inner lining of the uterus) by inserting a thin, flexible tube through the cervix and into the uterus. The tube is used to gently scrape a small amount of tissue from the endometrium and remove tissue samples. A pathologist views the tissue under a microscope to look for cancer cells.

Dilation and Curettage

A procedure also known as a D&C removes samples of tissue from the inner lining of the uterus. The cervix is dilated, and a curette (spoon-shaped instrument) is inserted into the uterus to remove tissue. The tissue samples are checked under a microscope for signs of disease.

Transvaginal Ultrasound

In addition to a general physical and pelvic exam, this imaging procedure (Chapter 6) along with a CT scan or MRI may also be used to detect cancer.

The prognosis (chance of recovery) and treatment options depend on the following:

- The stage of the cancer (whether it is in the endometrium only, involves the whole uterus, or has spread to other places in the body)
- How the cancer cells look under a microscope
- Whether the cancer cells are affected by progesterone

Surgical Options

Surgery is the most common treatment for endometrial cancer. The following surgical procedures may be used.

Total hysterectomy removes the uterus, including the cervix. If the uterus and cervix are taken out through the vagina, the operation is called a vaginal hysterectomy. If the uterus and cervix are taken out through a large incision (cut) in the abdomen, the operation is called a total abdominal hysterectomy. If the uterus and cervix are taken out through a small incision (cut) in the abdomen using a laparoscope, the operation is called a total laparoscopic hysterectomy.

A bilateral salpingo-oophorectomy removes both ovaries and fallopian tubes.

Radical hysterectomy surgery removes the uterus, cervix, and part of the vagina. The ovaries, fallopian tubes, or nearby lymph nodes may also be removed.

Even if the doctor removes all the cancer that can be seen at the time of the surgery, some patients may be given radiation therapy or hormone treatment after surgery to kill any cancer cells that are left. Treatment given after the surgery to lower the risk that the cancer will come back is called adjuvant therapy.

Robin Quivers: Aiming for a Cure

When listeners tune in to the *Howard Stern Show*, they expect the unexpected, and Robin Quivers has been a big part of that show for many years. But on the morning of September 9, 2013, an announcement that Stern's sidekick had been fighting cancer for the past fifteen months took most listeners by surprise.

In May 2012, while attending a wedding in Pittsburgh, Quivers

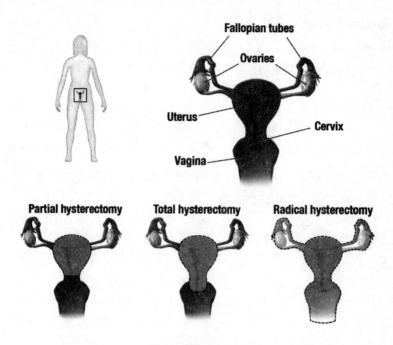

Types of Hysterectomy
Source: BruceBlaus (*commons.wikimedia.org/w/index.php?curid=44922548*)

wasn't able to pee. A doctor drained her bladder, but it happened again. A mass the size of a grapefruit was found in her uterus, and she received the diagnosis of endometrial cancer (cancer of the uterus).

Doctors initially told Robin that the outlook was bleak, that she would probably survive surgery but her quality of life would be diminished. They used words like *prolonging your life* instead of *curing you*. But Quivers met Dr. Carol Aghajanian at Memorial Sloan Kettering in New York City and Dr. David Agus from the University of Southern California in Los Angeles, who told her they not only could treat her, they were aiming for a cure.

Robin underwent two surgeries plus chemotherapy and radiation. She tolerated the chemo amazingly well and insisted on working throughout her treatment, which she did from her home studio for over a year, missing only three shows during that period.

In May 2013, doctors told Robin she was cancer-free.

Genetic Fingerprints of Uterine Cancers and New Approaches to Treatment

As we explained in Chapter 1 and elsewhere in this book, cancer is a disease of your DNA. The May 2, 2013, issue of the *New York Times* put it this way: "Cancer will increasingly be seen as a disease defined primarily by its genetic fingerprint rather than just by the organ where it originated."

The latest research is redefining uterine cancer into four different diseases based on different DNA fingerprints.

1. *Ultra-mutated endometrial cancers* have a critical defect in a gene called POLE that is responsible for "proofreading" errors in DNA. Loss of this proofreading function leads to the ultra-mutated state of the cancer cells.

2. *Hyper-mutated microsatellite endometrial cancers* have a defect in another DNA repair system that fixes mismatches among DNA strands. Microsatellites are stutters that occur in the language of DNA when the mismatches are not repaired. These tumors are said to possess microsatellite instability (MSI), which is characteristic of hereditary uterine cancers in patients with Lynch syndrome.

3. *Copy-number low endometrial cancers* have low mutation rates in their DNA but do have mutations in specific genes, such as PTEN, which is a tumor suppressor gene. When it loses its normal function, it enables cancers to form.

4. *Copy-number high serous cancers* also have low mutation rates,

but most have defects in a gene called TP53, also known as the "guardian of the genome." TP53 is the most frequently damaged gene in human cancers and is responsible for one type of hereditary breast cancer (Chapter 3).

A major advance in cancer treatment has been the development of immunotherapy drugs that harness the abilities of our immune systems to recognize cancers as foreign invaders of our bodies and mount a lethal attack on them. One of these drugs recently led to the seemingly miraculous cure of former President Jimmy Carter's malignant skin cancer (melanoma) that had spread to his liver and brain (Chapter 14).

Immunotherapy drugs work best on tumors that have highly disruptive genetic abnormalities, called high mutational burdens or loads. The ultra-mutated and hyper-mutated forms of uterine cancer seem to fall within this category, and, as of spring 2016, there is at least one clinical research trial that is recruiting patients to test new drugs.

You can find out more by going to *https://clinicaltrials.gov/*. Type in the search terms "endometrial immunotherapy." You can also track progress on our companion website *ReimaginingCancer.com*.

—————— MY JOURNEY ——————

I'm a fitness fanatic, so it took me a while to accept that I might have a problem with my body. My stomach wasn't right and I kept getting tired from my workouts, which never happened before. I went to a doctor, and after an MRI, a CT scan, ultrasound, and general exam, I was found to have a tumor and scheduled for surgery.

I had no history of cancer in my family and had always prided myself on eating right, exercising hard every day, and ingesting loads of supplements. So how could this happen to me? Well, it just did, and it turned out that I had uterine cancer, which after surgery left me facing menopause. I'm not as active as I was before, but I can still outrun my husband, and my kids are now kids again instead of freaked out little people worrying about their mother night and day. I've learned that no matter how healthy you *think* you are, you just might not be, and testing, even though it's not perfect, usually wins.

Rae (Cleveland, Ohio)

Uterine Sarcoma: Signs, Symptoms, and Risks

This is a rare tumor that forms in the muscles of the uterus and accounts for only about 3 percent of all uterine cancers. The following tumors are formed primarily from three distinct tissues:

1. *Carcinosarcomas* in the endometrium and in other organs of mullerian origin, which account for 40 to 50 percent of all uterine sarcomas.
2. *Leiomyosarcomas*, which originate in the myometrial muscle, with a peak incidence occurring at age fifty, and accounting for 30 percent of all uterine sarcomas.
3. *Sarcomas* arising in the endometrial stroma, with a peak incidence occurring before menopause for the low-grade tumors and after menopause for the high-grade tumors, which account for 15 percent of all uterine sarcomas.

The only documented causal factor in 10 to 25 percent of these tumors is prior pelvic radiation therapy. In the past, this was often administered for benign uterine bleeding, which had begun five to twenty-five years earlier.

An increased incidence of uterine sarcoma has also been associated with tamoxifen in the treatment of breast cancer. If you are taking this drug, have a pelvic exam every year and report any vaginal bleeding (other than menstrual bleeding) as soon as possible.

Check with your doctor if you have any of the following signs and symptoms:

- Bleeding that is not part of menstrual periods
- Bleeding after menopause
- A mass in the vagina
- Pain or a feeling of fullness in the abdomen
- Frequent urination

Side Effects of Uterine Cancer Treatments

After any hysterectomy, you will no longer have menstrual periods. If the ovaries are also removed during surgery, you will immediately go into menopause and may have menopausal symptoms such as hot flashes, night sweats, and/or vaginal itching or dryness.

Additional Side Effects of Surgery

- *Constipation:* This condition occurs in most women following a hysterectomy and can usually be controlled with a regimen of stool softeners, dietary fiber, and laxatives. Narcotic (opioid) pain medications taken after surgery can increase the likelihood of constipation.
- *Urinary retention:* The inability to pass urine can occur after vaginal hysterectomy. Urine can be drained using a catheter until retention resolves, usually within twenty-four to forty-eight hours.
- *Injury:* The urinary bladder, ureters (small tubes leading from the kidneys to the bladder), and large and small intestines, located in the lower abdomen and pelvis, and can be injured during a hysterectomy. Bladder injury occurs in 1 to 2 percent

of women who have a hysterectomy, while bowel injury occurs in less than 1 percent of women.

After surgery, normal physical activity can usually be resumed in four to eight weeks. Sexual desire and sexual intercourse are not typically affected by a hysterectomy. Some women, however, may have difficulty with intimacy because they are experiencing feelings of loss. If you feel that this may be true for you, speak to your doctor.

―――――――――― MY JOURNEY ――――――――――

For some reason, the second time around with uterine cancer was easier than the first, and most of that had to do with losing my hair all over again. The first time I was forced to go bald it felt like a novelty from hell, and I couldn't feel comfortable in my exercise classes or at home without a wig or a headscarf. When I went shopping, I felt better in a baseball cap, but I always dreaded being seen by someone I knew who would stop me to ask unintentionally invasive questions.

I had to admit at the time that after having long hair all my life, I was actually enjoying not needing to fuss with it at all, but still, I wasn't ready to admit that to the rest of the world.

The second time around, after surgery and what seemed like the longest chemo regimen I could imagine, I was comfortable right away losing my hair, and after it grew back, albeit much shorter, like a military man's buzz cut. I was happy looking like what my son called a "tough chick." I hardly felt tough at all; if anything, I felt horribly beaten up, but I no longer pined to put my hair in a ponytail or leave it loose over one shoulder. In fact, I plan on keeping my hair very short from here on. I still wear a wig sometimes—as a novelty—but from a much better place than hell.

Grace (Lincoln, Nebraska)

Radiation Therapy Side Effects

This therapy aimed at the pelvis may cause the following side effects:

- Diarrhea
- Rectal bleeding
- Incontinence
- Bladder irritation
- Changes in menstruation, such as stopping menstruating
- Symptoms of menopause, such as vaginal itching, burning, and dryness
- Shortening of the vagina
- Pain with intercourse

Women may be advised not to have intercourse during treatment; however, most can resume sexual activity within a few weeks after treatment ends.

> **NOTE to PATIENT:**
> Anything that increases our risk of getting a
> disease is called a risk factor,
> which does not mean that we will get cancer—
> just as not having risk factors doesn't mean that we will not.
> Talk with your doctor if you think you may be at risk.

KEY POINTS TO REMEMBER

✓ Cancer of the endometrium is the most common cancer of the female reproductive organs.

✓ The average chance of a woman being diagnosed with this cancer during her lifetime is about one in thirty-seven.

✓ Most uterine cancers start in the endometrium, which forms the inner lining of the uterus.

✓ Women with Lynch syndrome have a greatly elevated risk of developing colon and endometrial cancers.

✓ Know your family history and see a genetic counselor if you think that any type of cancer runs in your family.

✓ Being exposed to estrogen increases a woman's risk of developing endometrial cancer.

✓ Tamoxifen is used to prevent breast cancer in women who are at high risk for the disease.

✓ Because endometrial cancer begins inside the uterus, it does not usually show up in the results of a Pap test.

✓ Surgery is the most common treatment for endometrial cancer.

✓ DNA research is showing that endometrial cancer is really four different diseases.

✓ Reimagining uterine cancer may lead to new treatments.

✓ After any hysterectomy, you will no longer have menstrual periods.

✓ Most women can resume sexual activity within a few weeks after treatment ends.

POEM TO MY UTERUS

you uterus
you have been patient
as a sock
while i have slippered into you
my dead and living children
now
they want to cut you out
stocking i will not need
where i am going
where am i going
old girl
without you
uterus
my bloody print
my estrogen kitchen
my black bag of desire
where can i go
barefoot
without you
where can you go
without me

—Lucille Clifton (1936–2010)
from *Collected Poems of Lucille Clifton*

8 RAISING AWARENESS: Cancer of the Cervix

Most doctors will not investigate thoroughly.
There's this idea that if you hear galloping and you
see a horse, you shouldn't look for a zebra.
That's great and all, until you realize
that there really was a zebra.
If we could spot the zebras—
if we could detect cancers early—
95 percent of people would be cured.
Stage I, that's the cure.

—Fran Drescher, as told to *brainworldmagazine.com*

New News

Cervical cancer is almost always caused by an infection of the cervix with human papillomavirus (HPV), which is one of the most common sexually transmitted infections in the United States. In fact, at some point in their lives, more than half of sexually active people are infected with one or more types of HPV.

Cervical cancer is highly preventable in most Western countries because of good screening tests and a vaccine that prevents HPV infections. When cervical cancer is found early, it is highly treatable and associated with long survival and good quality of life.

Basic Anatomy and Function

The cervix is the lower, narrow end of the uterus (Chapter 7) and leads from the uterus to the vagina (birth canal).

In a nonpregnant woman, the cervix is between two and three centimeters long and its shape is cylindrical. A narrow, central cervical canal runs along its entire length, connecting the uterine cavity and the opening of the vagina. The opening into the uterus is called the internal os and the opening into the vagina is called the external os.

The lower end of the cervix, called the ectocervix, bulges through the front wall of the vagina. The portion of the cervix that lies between the uterus and the vagina is called the endocervix. The endocervical canal, which passes through the cervix, is lined with a single layer of column-shaped cells that are sometimes sampled for diagnosis by a procedure called endocervical curettage (described later in this chapter). The ectocervix is made up of multiple layers of cells topped with a scale-like surface layer similar to that of the vagina. These are the cells sampled during a Pap smear.

Many glands in the endocervix produce mucus. The consistency of the cervical mucus can vary quite a bit over the course of a menstrual cycle. These changes allow it to function either as a barrier or a transport medium to sperm, optimizing the correct time for fertilization of an egg.

Mid-cycle—when an egg is about to be released—under the influence of high estrogen levels, the mucus is thin and watery to allow sperm to enter the uterus. Its composition is more alkaline, which is

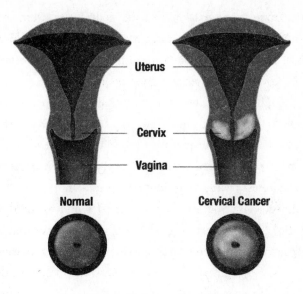

Anatomy of the Cervix, Cervical Cancer
Source: © Alila07 | *Dreamstime.com*

more hospitable to sperm. At other times in the cycle, the mucus is thick and more acidic due to the effects of progesterone. This mucus acts as a barrier to sperm, preventing them from entering the uterus.

Defining Cervical Cancer and Screening

There are two main types of cervical cancer. Squamous cell carcinoma begins in the thin, flat cells that line the cervix. Adenocarcinoma begins in cervical glands that produce mucus and other fluids.

According to American Cancer Society's estimates,[13] approximately 12,900 new cases of invasive cervical cancer were diagnosed in the United States in 2015, and about 4,100 women died from the disease.

---

13. *http://www.cancer.org/cancer/cervicalcancer/detailedguide/cervical-cancer-key-statistics*

Worldwide, more than half a million women are diagnosed with cervical cancer every year, and more than a quarter million die from the disease.

Cervical cancer used to be the leading cause of cancer death for women in the United States. But over the last forty years, the death rate has gone down by more than 50 percent. The main reason for this change is the increased use of the Pap test, or vaginal smear, that can detect precancerous changes as well as diagnose cervical cancer.

The Pap test is named after Dr. Georgios Papanicolaou, who invented this test, which was first publicized in 1946. For many decades, a yearly Pap test was a routine part of a woman's annual gynecologic (GYN) exam. The guidelines for testing changed in 2012, and we'll describe the current recommendations later in this chapter.

Jade Goody: A Cancer Fight Instructs a Nation

By her mid twenties, Jade Goody was a reality show star in England, appearing on several shows, including the UK version of *Big Brother* and *Celebrity Big Brother*, as well as an Indian version, called *Bigg Boss*. In August 2008, shortly after filming began for *Bigg Boss*, Jade was diagnosed with cervical cancer. She was only twenty-seven years old.

Ms. Goody underwent a radical hysterectomy followed by radiation therapy and chemotherapy. By October, the cancer had spread to her liver and intestines, and she underwent emergency surgery to remove a tumor in her abdomen. Despite her illness, Jade regularly appeared in public—often bald—and participated in two documentaries: *Living with Jade Goody*, and *Jade's Cancer Battle*. She even wrote an autobiography entitled *Jade: Catch a Falling Star*.

Coverage of her illness by British media remained heavy throughout her illnesses. From the time her diagnosis was first reported in August 2008 until ten weeks after her death, over 1,200 articles about her case appeared in numerous newspapers. Awareness of Goody's disease caused remarkable spikes in Internet searches for information on cervical cancer, leading to the definition of the Jade Goody Effect. These sharp increases in search engine traffic investigating specific diseases/medical conditions demonstrate once again the power a celebrity can have in calling attention to underreported diseases and the role early detection and prevention can play in diminishing the harm these conditions create.

Jade Goody died in her sleep in March 2009. Her most important legacy was the effect her public cancer battle had on cervical cancer awareness, prevention, and screening. According to Cancer Research UK, Jade's story "raised awareness of cervical cancer, which has led to hundreds of thousands of people contacting Cancer Research UK for information on the disease, as the number of hits to our website, *CancerHelp.org* shows. Her legacy will be to help save lives."

Current Guidelines for Screening in the United States

Having an annual Pap test to screen for early cervical cancer is no longer recommended by leading medical organizations, such as the American Cancer Society (ACS) and the U.S. Preventative Services Task Force (USPSTF).

Current recommendations are the following:

- *No screening for women younger than twenty-one.* Cervical cancer is rare in young women, and screening can lead to unnecessary follow-up tests or treatments as well as psychological stress.
- *For women twenty-one to sixty-five-years old,* a Pap smear should be done every three years—or—a Pap smear in combination with HPV testing every five years.
- *No screening for women over sixty-five* unless they are at high risk or lack prior screening data.

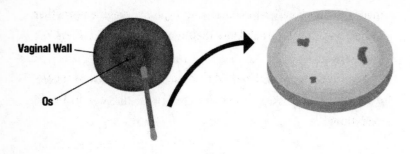

Pap Smear
Source: Joshua Abbas (*123rf.com*)

Signs and Symptoms

Early cervical cancer may not exhibit signs or symptoms. When it does, these can include vaginal bleeding (including bleeding after sexual intercourse), unusual vaginal discharge, pelvic pain, or pain during sexual intercourse.

─────────── **MY JOURNEY** ───────────

Abnormalities? I wondered what that could mean, especially because I heard that word used during my first cervical screening. I was only twenty-eight, and I didn't know anything at all about cancer. I didn't even know enough to be freaked out, and when I found out how common it is, I just said, "Bring it on! Let's get this over with."

If only it had been that easy!

But while I saw many women struggling, I was fortunate to have so much love in my corner. After a radical hysterectomy, which removed my womb and lymph glands, I had a tough recovery. A few weeks later, I was feeling more like myself, even though I knew I would never be a whole woman again, as in capable of having children. My son made that much easier, of course, and I cannot imagine how other women go through this and lose the chance to have kids. That's just plain cruel.

I survived because of early detection, and I want all women—especially young ones—to realize that early screening means everything!

Yolanda (Baton Rouge, Louisiana)

How Is Cervical Cancer Diagnosed?

Because we now know that a sexually transmitted virus called HPV (discussed in this chapter) causes cervical cancer, testing for this virus is often done in conjunction with the Pap smear. It's called a "smear" because cells collected from a swab of the cervix are smeared onto a glass slide for examination under a microscope.

Hispanic women or those of Native American ancestry have a higher frequency of cervical cancer than women from other racial or ethnic groups. Death rates in African American women remain higher than women of any other racial or ethnic group in the United States.

Yvette Wilson: "Cancer Sucks!"

An actress best known for her role as Andell Wilkerson on UPN's *Moesha* and its spinoff *The Parkers*, Yvette Wilson also appeared in a number of movies, including *House Party 2, House Party 3, Friday*, and on Russell Simmons's *Def Comedy Jam*.

After her initial treatment for cervical cancer, she had "an extended retreat" from the disease. However, when the cancer returned, it did so very aggressively. Besides dealing with a stage IV re-diagnosis, Wilson was also plagued by kidney failure.

Before her death, a friend and fellow stage IV cancer survivor, Jeffrey Pittle, created a fund called Yvette Wilson's Cancer Sucks Fund to raise money for her medical treatment. Unfortunately, she passed away in June 2012 at the age of forty-eight.

African American Women and Cervical Cancer

Wilson's cancer story calls attention to the fact that despite an overall decrease in the incidence of cervical cancer, African American women continue to have higher mortality rates than any other group.

What's the reason for this disparity? Some people suggest that the difference is socioeconomic because many black women have less access to screening and follow-up care. But the real answer may be biological. One recent study looked at HPV infections of women who attended college in South Carolina.[14] Every six months, women enrolled in the study received Pap smears and were also tested for HPV. Researchers found essentially no difference in the incidence of new HPV infections between black and white women. But the African American women were more likely to test positive for high-risk HPV types, and they seemed to have more difficulty clearing those infections. The median length of infection in white women was about twelve months, compared with nineteen months in black women. The reasons for this slower clearance remain unknown and are under further investigation.

Because HPV infection can lead to an abnormal Pap smear, researchers compared the Pap smears and found that African American women were almost two times more likely to have abnormal results than white women.

---

14. Carolyn E. Banister, Amy R. Messersmith, Hrishikesh Chakraborty, Yinding Wang, Lisa B. Spiryda, Saundra H. Glover, Lucia Pirisi, and Kim E. Creek, "HPV prevalence at enrollment and baseline results from the Carolina Women's Care Study, a longitudinal study of HPV persistence in women of college age," *International Journal of Women's Health* 5 (2013): 379–88.

———————————— MY JOURNEY ————————————

After I had my cervix removed—along with my uterus, ovaries, and fallopian tubes—I was overwhelmed with pain, fear, and confusion about what was ahead and how I could ever deal with any of it. Honestly, I wanted to give up, and if it weren't for my family and the support of an amazing oncology social worker, I probably wouldn't have made it. Now, with lots of what people call alternative therapies, I still have a large, ugly scar, but the rest of me is healing pretty well. Fixing my diet, taking yoga classes, and attending group support classes every week have made a world of difference for me. Everything I do to take attention off of my downside gives me hope, and that sustains me each day. So that scar just reminds me of what I have been through, how far I have come, and how far I hope to still be going.

Rachel (Toronto, Canada)

What You Need to Know About Cervical Cancer and HPV

HPV is a small DNA virus that contains only eight genes and is a group of more than 150 related viruses. More than forty of them can be easily spread through direct skin-to-skin contact during vaginal, anal, and oral sex. Sexually transmitted HPVs fall into two categories: low-risk HPV and high-risk HPV.

Low-risk HPVs do not cause cancer but can cause skin warts (technically known as condylomata acuminata) on or around the genitals or anus. For example, HPV-6 and HPV-11 cause 90 percent of all genital warts.

High-risk HPVs are oncogenic, literally meaning "cancer causing." At least a dozen high-risk HPV types have been identified. Two of these, HPV types 16 and 18 (HPV-16, HPV-18), are responsible for the majority of HPV-caused cancers.

High-risk HPV infection accounts for approximately 5 percent of all cancers worldwide. It's important to know that most high-risk HPV infections occur without any symptoms, go away within one to two years, and do not cause cancer. These transient infections may cause cytological abnormalities (abnormal appearance of cervical cells from a Pap smear) that go away on their own.

Some HPV infections, however, can persist for many years. Persistent infections with high-risk HPV types can lead to more serious cytological abnormalities or lesions that if untreated may progress to cancer.

How High-Risk HPVs Cause Cancer

HPVs infect squamous cells. Cancers of these cells are called squamous cell carcinomas (or SCC). Squamous (pronounced "skway-mus") cells are flat and organized in layers and cover some inside and outside surfaces of the body, including the skin, mouth, tongue, throat, genital tract, and the anus. HPVs are not thought to enter the bloodstream; therefore, an HPV infection in one part of the body will not cause an infection in another part of the body.

Once an HPV enters a cell, the viral genes begin to make proteins. Some of these proteins made by high-risk HPVs interfere with normal functions in the cell, enabling the cell to grow in an uncontrolled manner and avoid cell death.

Many times these infected cells are recognized by the immune system and eliminated. In other words, the infection is transient. Sometimes, however, these infected cells are not destroyed and a persistent infection results. As the persistently infected cells continue to grow, they may develop mutations that promote even more cell growth, leading to the formation of a precancerous lesion that can eventually become a malignant tumor.

Researchers believe that it can take between ten and thirty years from the time of an initial HPV infection until a tumor forms. However, precancerous growths do not always lead to cancer, but there's about a fifty-fifty chance they will. This means that women with persistent infections, some of which can last from twenty to thirty years, are considerably more vulnerable to getting cancer later in their lives.

Nearly all cervical cancers are caused by HPV infections, with just two HPV types, 16 and 18, responsible for about 70 percent of all cases. A study at Duke University found that although African American women had infections with HPV types 16 and 18, these types were found only 50 percent of the time. Other types, especially types 33, 35, 58, and 68, were more common. This finding may be important in terms of HPV vaccination.

HPV also causes anal cancer, with about 85 percent of all cases caused by HPV. Types 16 and 18 have also been found to cause nearly half of vaginal, vulvar, and penile cancers.

Most recently, HPV infections have been found to cause cancer of the oropharynx, which is the middle part of the throat including the soft palate, the base of the tongue, and the tonsils. In the United States, more than half of the cancers diagnosed in the oropharynx are linked to HPV-16.

The incidence of HPV-associated oropharyngeal cancer has increased during the past twenty years, especially among men. Michael Douglas famously said that oral sex caused his throat cancer. It has been estimated that by 2020, HPV will cause more oropharyngeal cancers than cervical cancers in the United States.

The good news is that there are highly effective vaccines now available to prevent HPV infection. You can find more about vaccines later in this chapter.

Human papilloma virus (HPV)

Sexually transmitted HPV infections are common and often asymptomatic, untreated cases in women are the main cause of cervical cancer

▶ A sexually transmitted virus that causes cancer

▶ More than 100 types of HPV have been found so far

▶ 15 have been identified as putting women at high risk for cervical cancer

Cervical Cancer

1 Virus in cervix enters cells through microabrasions

Infects cells

Several weeks later

2 HPV replicates

90 percent of cases heal within two years

Infection spreads

10-30 years later

3 0.8 percent of cases develop cancer

HPV invades deeper layer of tissues and turns cancerous

Source: Nobel/FDA

Human Papilloma Virus (HPV)
Source: AFP (used with permission)

––––––––––––––––– MY JOURNEY –––––––––––––––––

I am fifty-two years old, married to my high school sweetheart, and the mother of three kids. Last year, during a routine check-up, I told my doc that something in my gut didn't feel right, so she did a biopsy and HPV test. I was subsequently diagnosed with cervical adenocarcinoma. We were both extremely surprised because none of the usual risk factors associated with this type of cancer applied to me, like multiple partners (remember, I married my childhood love), smoking (never!), or long-term use of oral birth control (Catholic!). My weight has never been an issue, and my exams and Pap smears have always come back negative. I had no reason to suspect any-thing, and that gut feeling only came about because I had recently gone through what they told me was perimenopause, which had me doubting everything about my changing body.

After a long recovery from major surgery, I am facing continual testing for the next five years until I can be considered free of cancer, in other words—cured.

I know how lucky I am that it was found early, but I wonder if I could have avoided this whole ordeal if a positive HPV test *before* my diagnosis had waved the red flag. Now, because of the HPV vaccine, most, if not all, of the younger generation should never experience what I had to go through.

Alene (Phoenix, Arizona)

Marissa Jaret-Minokur:
The Importance of HPV Testing

Best known for her performance as Tracy Turnblad in the Broadway musical *Hairspray*, Marissa Jaret-Minokur won the Tony Award for Best Leading Actress in a Musical in 2003. But in 2001, during the rehearsal period for *Hairspray*, Marissa found out that a routine Pap test—after years of normal tests—was positive for cervical cancer. She was twenty-eight years old.

"I was scheduled to have a hysterectomy right after the final rehearsal for *Hairspray*. Because the show hadn't started its run on Broadway yet, I was afraid to tell anyone other than my immediate family that I had cancer. I didn't want to jeopardize my opportunity to play the biggest role of my life, or to be known as 'the cancer girl.'"[15]

Marissa underwent a hysterectomy. Fortunately, the surgeons were able to save her ovaries. At the time, Marissa was thinking more about surviving than having children. But she now knows how fortunate she was, because in 2008, she had a son, Zev, via a surrogate.

"My brush with cancer put everything into perspective, and made me realize I had to take charge of my life and my health. Now I want to use that newfound 'empowerment' to help other women do the same. I'm a lot more educated today, and I know that the Pap sometimes doesn't catch abnormal cells until the cancer is already there. That was the case for me. I also now realize that we know the cause of cervical cancer, HPV, and that there is a test that can detect it. Getting the HPV test along with a Pap helps make sure you know if you're at risk early, before it's too late."

Can Immunization Prevent Cancer?

The answer is a resounding *yes!* Cervical cancer is one of the few cancers whose primary cause can be linked to a specific virus—HPV— and there are now three FDA-approved vaccines to prevent HPV infection: Gardasil, Gardasil 9, and Cervarix.

---

15. *https://web.archive.org/web/20080619074930/http://www.thehpvtest.com/cervical-cancer-survivor -stories-marissa-jaret-winokur.html?terms=Winokur*

Widespread vaccination with Cervarix or Gardasil has the potential to reduce cervical cancer incidence around the world by as much as two-thirds, while Gardasil 9 could prevent an even higher proportion. In addition, the vaccines can reduce the need for medical care, biopsies, and invasive procedures associated with follow-up from abnormal cervical screening. Together, this could reduce healthcare costs and anxieties related to follow-up procedures.

Like other immunizations that guard against viral infections, HPV vaccines stimulate the body to produce antibodies that, in future encounters with HPV, bind to the virus and prevent it from infecting cells. The current HPV vaccines are based on virus-like particles (VLPs) that are formed by HPV surface components. VLPs are not infectious because they lack the virus's DNA. However, they closely resemble the natural virus, and antibodies against the VLPs also have activity against the natural virus. VLPs are strongly immunogenic, which means that they induce high levels of antibody production by the body. This makes the vaccines highly effective.

HPV vaccines are very effective in preventing infection with the types of HPV they target but are most effective when they are given *before* any initial exposure to the virus—before an individual begins to engage in sexual activity. This is why the Advisory Committee on Immunization Practices (ACIP)[16] recommends that routine HPV vaccinations begin at age eleven or twelve. The vaccination series can safely be started as young as nine. They also recommend vaccination of females between thirteen and twenty-six years old and of males aged thirteen to twenty-one who have not been vaccinated previously or who have not completed the complete, three-dose vaccination series.

---

16. ACIP is a group of fifteen medical and public health experts that develops recommendations on how to use vaccines to control diseases in the United States.

Although HPV vaccines are safe when given to people who are already infected with HPV, the vaccines do not treat infection. They provide maximum benefit if a person receives them before he or she is sexually active.

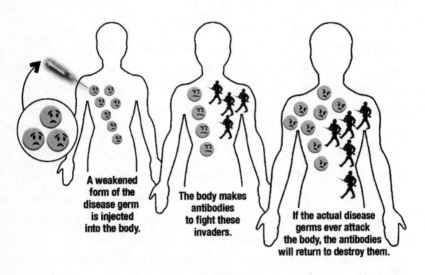

How a Vaccine Works
Source: Centers for Disease Control

Three HPV Vaccines: What's the Difference?

All three vaccines—Gardasil, Gardasil 9, and Cervarix—prevent infections with HPV types 16 and 18, two high-risk HPVs that cause about 70 percent of cervical cancers.

Gardasil also prevents infection with HPV types 6 and 11, which cause 90 percent of genital warts. Gardasil 9 is the newest HPV vaccine. It prevents infection with the same four HPV types as Gardasil, plus five additional high-risk HPV types (31, 33, 45, 52, and 58).

The FDA approved Gardasil and Gardasil 9 for use in girls and women ages nine through twenty-six for the prevention of HPV-caused cervical, vulvar, vaginal, and anal cancers, precancerous cervical, vaginal, and anal conditions, as well as genital warts. Cervarix is approved for use in females ages nine to twenty-six for the prevention of cervical cancer.

All three HPV vaccines are designed to be dispensed in three shots over a six-month period. The second shot is given one or two months after the first shot, and the third shot is given six months after the first shot.

Before any vaccine is approved for use, the FDA must determine that it is both safe and effective. All three HPV vaccines have been tested in tens of thousands of people in the United States and many other countries. Thus far, the vaccines have shown no evidence of any serious side effects. The most common problems have been brief soreness and other local symptoms at the injection site. These problems are similar to those commonly experienced with other vaccines.

The vaccines have not been sufficiently tested during pregnancy and therefore should not be used by pregnant women.

Vaccinations and Screening

If you've been vaccinated, you still need to be screened for cervical cancer. This is because these vaccines do not protect against all HPV types that can cause cancer; therefore, screening continues to be an essential method for detecting precancerous changes in cervical cells *before* they develop into cancer. In addition, cervical screening tests—the HPV DNA test alone or the HPV and Pap test together, also known as co-testing—are critically important for women who have not been vaccinated or who are already infected with HPV.

As more young women become immunized, there could be future changes in screening recommendations for vaccinated women.

────────────── MY JOURNEY ──────────────

If I could, I would tell everyone that HPV is a common infection and almost all of us get it at one point or another. In fact, by the time women turn fifty years old, the HPV virus will infect nearly 80 percent of women. The answer to this is quite simple: women need to become better informed! They need to engage their doctors! They need to get the facts and be proactive! It's our responsibility to protect ourselves—and our families.

Carol (St. Paul, Minnesota)

What About Abnormal Pap Smears?

About one in twenty women have abnormal results after a cervical screening test. Not all of these cases are cancer or precancer. If your Pap smear is abnormal and you've not had an HPV test, your gynecologist may recommend one, or perhaps just repeat the Pap smear on your next office visit. If your gynecologist suspects cancer, he or she may perform the following procedures:

- *Endocervical curettage:* A procedure to collect cells or tissue from the cervical canal using a curette (spoon-shaped instrument). Tissue samples are checked under a microscope for signs of cancer. This procedure is sometimes done at the same time as a colposcopy.
- *Colposcopy:* A procedure in which a colposcope (a lighted, magnifying instrument) is used to check the vagina and cervix for abnormal areas. Tissue samples may be taken using a curette or a brush and checked under a microscope for signs of disease.
- *Biopsy:* A sample of tissue is cut from the cervix and viewed under a microscope by a pathologist to check for signs of

cancer. A biopsy that removes only a small amount of tissue is usually done in the doctor's office. A woman may need to go to a hospital for a cervical cone biopsy (removal of a larger, cone-shaped sample of cervical tissue).

• A pathologist will examine the removed tissue to see if cancer is present and how deeply it may have spread. If you ask to read your pathology report, you might see terms like SISCCA, which stands for superficially invasive squamous cell carcinoma. This diagnosis means that the cone biopsy (described later) was curative and you'll probably need no further treatment.

Treatment Options

There are different types of treatment for patients with cervical cancer. Determining the most appropriate treatment will depend on the stage of the cancer, the specific type of cervical cancer, the patient's age, and her desire to have children.

Surgery

This traditional method is commonly used to treat cervical cancer and also to stage the extent of the disease. The following procedures may be used:

Conization (also known as a cone biopsy) is a procedure to remove a cone-shaped piece of tissue from the cervix and cervical canal. The procedure may be used to diagnose/treat cervical cancer. Conization (surgery) may be done using one of the following procedures:

Cold-knife conization uses a scalpel (sharp knife) to remove abnormal tissue or cancer.

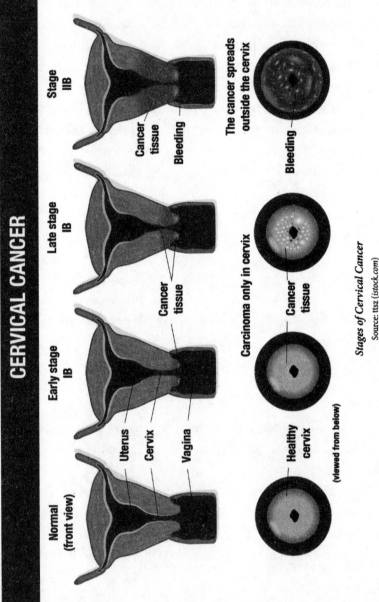

Stages of Cervical Cancer
Source: ttsz (istock.com)

Loop electrosurgical excision procedure (LEEP) passes an electrical current through a thin wire loop (as a knife) to remove abnormal tissue or cancer.

Laser surgery uses a laser beam (a narrow beam of intense light) as a knife to make bloodless cuts in tissue or to remove a surface lesion such as a tumor.

The type of conization procedure used depends on where the cancer cells are in the cervix and the specific type of cervical cancer.

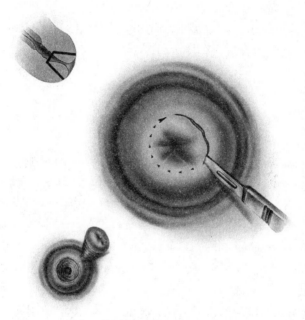

Conization Procedure
Source: Judith Glick Enrenthal (*istock.com*)

In a total hysterectomy, a surgeon removes the entire uterus, including the cervix. This can be done one of several ways:

Vaginal hysterectomy, through the vagina.

Total abdominal hysterectomy, through an incision in the
   abdomen.
Total laparoscopic hysterectomy, through several small incisions
   in the abdomen using a laparoscope (possibly performed
   with the assistance of a surgical robot).

Depending on the spread of the cancer, other procedures, such as a
radical hysterectomy and modified radical hysterectomy, may be done.
In these procedures, in addition to removing the uterus and cervix,
part of the vagina and local ligaments and tissues are also removed.
Depending on the particular pathology of the patient, the ovaries,
fallopian tubes, and/or nearby lymph nodes may also be removed.

Can I Start a Family?

Michelle L. Whitlock was twenty-six years old—fit as a fiddle,
zooming in her career, and enjoying a budding romance—when she
was diagnosed with cervical cancer. Since she wanted to someday start
a family, she opted for a relatively new procedure called a trachelectomy, in which her cervix was removed but her uterus remained. This
surgery gives women about a 50 percent chance of conceiving in the
future, and in Michelle's case, it led her into remission.

Two years later, just after her boyfriend proposed, Michelle discovered that the cancer was back . . . and had spread, necessitating a
hysterectomy to save her life. Just before undergoing surgery, Michelle
found a fertility clinic to create frozen embryos, and she and her fiancé
went to Jamaica to get married at the beach. With the aid of a gestational host, also known as a surrogate mother, Michelle had a healthy
baby girl.

"I don't regret not having a hysterectomy right away," Michelle
says. "That decision bought me two years to fall in love, get married,

and have a plan. So I didn't see that as a mistake—I saw it as an opportunity."

Michelle's 2011 book, *How I Lost My Uterus and Found My Voice: A Memoir of Love, Hope, and Empowerment*, explores her fight to live, love, and have children. "I want to help other women know there is life after cancer and it can be wonderful. Be empowered, do your own research, and ask the tough questions. As patients, we have to remember to use doctors as our partners, but to still speak up and be part of the treatment plan. Without that, I wouldn't have this precious little angel."

Radiation Therapy

Radiation therapy may be used on its own when treating cervical cancer or in combination with surgery/chemotherapy. It uses high-energy X-rays or other types of radiation to kill cancer cells or keep them from growing.

The three types of radiation therapy most often used are presented here:

1. *External* radiation therapy uses a machine outside the body to send radiation toward the specific location of the cancer.
2. *Internal* radiation therapy uses a radioactive substance sealed in needles, seeds, wires, or catheters that are placed directly into or near the cancer. The precise manner on which the radiation is given depends on the type and stage of the cancer being treated.
3. *Intensity-modulated* radiation therapy (IMRT) is a type of three-dimensional (3-D) radiation therapy that uses a computer to make pictures of the size and shape of the tumor. Thin beams of radiation of different intensities (strengths) are

aimed at the tumor from many angles. This type of radiation therapy causes less damage to healthy tissue near the tumor.

Chemotherapy and Targeted Therapy

Despite tremendous advances in the prevention of cervical cancer and screening for early stage disease, approximately 5 percent of women who are diagnosed with cervical cancer in North America have advanced, metastatic (stage IV) disease.

Patients like these are usually treated with a combination of therapies that include two chemotherapy drugs (cisplatin and paclitaxel) plus a targeted drug called bevacizumab (Avastin) that "starves" tumors of their blood supplies.

--------- MY JOURNEY ---------

Any woman dealing with a cancer diagnosis in her lower body, whether it's cervical, uterine, vaginal, etc., probably has one big question pop up in her mind out of all her other concerns, and even if she doesn't say it out loud, it's got to be on her mind: Will I ever be able to have sexual intercourse again?

Between the surgery and the radiation and what those do to the body, you just don't know what's happening to your body, much less the psychological twist all of this puts you through. Should I start grieving now for the loss of this fundamental part of my life? Will my capability and drive ever return? These are really hard things to discuss with a spouse, let alone your doctor. From my own experience, if you don't, you're leaving yourself on an island of doubt, and that's a terrible place to be. Speak up! It's hard to talk about, but even harder to live in silence.

Beth (New York, New York)

Side Effects of Cervical Cancer Treatments

Surgery: Side effects or possible complications of surgery are related to how extensive an operation a patient undergoes. Surgical treatment for cervical cancer may cause cramping, vaginal bleeding, or produce a watery discharge.

Radiation therapy: If you have received external radiation, it is common to lose hair in the treated area and for the skin to become red, dry, tender, and itchy. There may also be permanent darkening or "bronzing" of the skin in the treated area.

The vagina can become narrower and less flexible, which can make intercourse painful. You may be taught how to use a vaginal dilator to help minimize these problems. A dilator is a tube-shaped device that is designed to gently stretch the vagina. Used with a lubricant, it is inserted into the vagina for short periods of time. Usually, women are told not to have intercourse during radiation therapy or while an implant is in place. However, most women can have sexual relations within a few weeks after treatment ends.

Drug Therapy: Side effects of cisplatin can include nausea and vomiting, low blood counts, and kidney problems. Side effects of paclitaxel can include edema, rashes, and hypersensitivity reactions that may result in low blood pressure and shortness of breath. Patients being treated with bevacizumab (Avastin) can experience problems with wound healing and bleeding, which sometimes can be severe. This drug can also cause holes (perforations) in the gastrointestinal tract.

For more information on the general risks and side effects of cancer surgery, radiation, chemotherapy, and other assorted drug therapies, please see Chapter 10.

KEY POINTS TO REMEMBER

✓ Cervical cancer is almost always caused by persistent infection of the cervix with human papillomavirus (HPV).

✓ HPV infection is the most common sexually transmitted disease in the United States.

✓ Highly effective vaccines are now available to prevent HPV infection and are recommended for girls and boys *before* they become sexually active.

✓ HPV can also cause cancers of the penis and oral cavity (mouth, tongue, tonsils) and larynx (voice box).

✓ If you've been vaccinated, you still need to be screened for cervical cancer.

✓ Early cervical cancer may not cause signs or symptoms.

✓ Women between the ages of twenty-one and sixty-five should have a Pap smear every three years or a Pap smear in combination with HPV testing every five years.

✓ Hispanic women or those of Native American ancestry have a higher frequency of cervical cancer than women from other racial or ethnic groups.

✓ When cervical cancer is found early, it is highly treatable.

✓ Determining the most appropriate treatment will depend on the stage of the cancer, the specific type of cervical cancer, the patient's age, and her desire to have children.

Farewell to Hair

I stood outside on a windy day
and ran my fingers through my hair.
Long strands of silky threads
blew across the lawn.
They glistened in the sun,
too many to count.

I imagined a nest,
lined with my mane,
woven by a mama bird.
The babies nestled,
snug inside,
warmed by my fallen tresses.

Now on the wintry nights,
when my head is cold,
I pull my wool cap
over my ears and smile
as I dream of baby birds
sleeping in my hair.

—Terri Hanson
the cancer poetry project

9 VaIN CANCERS AND DES DAUGHTERS: Understanding Cancers of the Vagina and Vulva

I know how scary cancer diagnosis can be—it was for me.
But I beat cancer,
and I know we can turn tears of sorrow into
tears of joy if we support this movement.

—Sofia Vergara

The Exception, Not the Rule

Cancers of the vagina and vulva are much less common than other gynecologic cancers, also know as "below the belt" cancers. The Centers for Disease Control and Prevention (CDC) reports that they account for 6 to 7 percent of all gynecologic cancers diagnosed in the United States, with an estimated 1,000 women diagnosed with vaginal cancer and 3,500 women with vulvar cancer each year.

In the United States, vulvar cancer accounts for about 4 percent of cancers of the female reproductive organs, which represent less than 1 percent of all cancers in women. In the United States, women have a 1 in 333 chance of developing vulvar cancer at some point in their lifetimes. The American Cancer Society projected approximately 5,150 cases of vulvar cancer would be diagnosed last year, and of those estimates about 1,080 women would not survive.

Basic Anatomy and Function

The vagina is the canal leading from the cervix, the opening of uterus (Chapter 8), to the outside of the body. During a natural birth, a baby leaves the mother's body through the vagina, which is also often referred to as the birth canal.

The vulva is made up of multiple parts, which include the following:

- Inner and outer lips of the vagina
- Clitoris (sensitive tissue between the lips)
- Opening of the vagina and its glands
- Mons pubis (rounded area in front of pubic bones, becomes covered with hair at puberty)
- Perineum (the area between the vulva and the anus)

Vaginal Cancers

Vaginal cancer refers to a disease that occurs when malignant (cancer) cells form in the vagina. Carcinomas of the vagina are uncommon tumors comprising only about 1 percent of the cancers that arise in the female genital system. There are two main types of vaginal cancer.

1. *Squamous cell carcinoma* (SCC) is the most common type of vaginal cancer, accounting for approximately 85 percent of

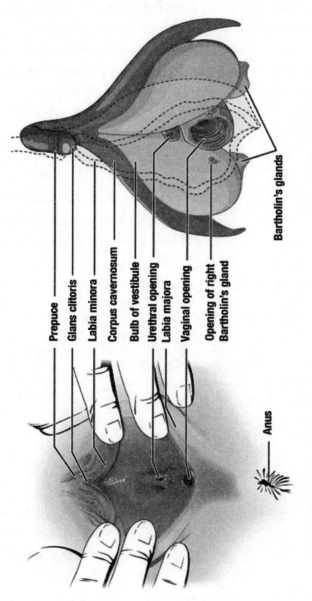

Prepuce
Glans clitoris
Labia minora
Corpus cavernosum
Bulb of vestibule
Urethral opening
Labia majora
Vaginal opening
Opening of right
Bartholin's gland

Bartholin's glands

Anus

Vulva: External anterior view

Vulva: Internal anteriolateral view

Anatomy of the Vagina and Vulva

Source: OpenStax College—Anatomy & Physiology, Connexions Web site.
http://cnx.org/content/col11496/1.6/, Jun 19, 2013., CC BY 3.0, https://commons.wikimedia.org/w/index.php?curid=30148635

vaginal cancer cases. This cancer forms in squamous cells—
thin, flat cells that line the vagina. These cancers are caused
by chronic infection with human papillomavirus or HPV
(Chapter 8 and later in this chapter). Squamous cell vaginal
cancer spreads slowly and usually stays near the vagina but
may spread to the lungs, liver, or bone.

2. *Adenocarcinoma* begins in glandular (secretory) cells that line
the vagina and release mucus. Approximately 5 to 10 percent
of cases of vaginal cancers are adenocarcinomas. They are
more likely than SCC to spread to the lymph nodes and distant organs, such as the lungs. A rare type of adenocarcinoma
is linked to exposure to diethylstilbestrol (DES) before birth.
Adenocarcinomas that are not linked with DES exposure are
most common in women after menopause. A pathologist
diagnoses these cancers after a gynecologist obtains a biopsy
of the suspected cancer.

Risk Factors for Vaginal Cancer

Although they can vary by each individual, risk factors for vaginal
cancer include the following:

- Age sixty or older.
- Persistent human papillomavirus (HPV) infection (Chapter 8)
- Exposure to DES while in the mother's womb (Note: Some
  of these daughters develop a rare form of vaginal cancer called
  clear cell adenocarcinoma.)
- History of abnormal cells in the cervix (abnormal Pap smear)
  or cervical cancer
- History of abnormal cells in the uterus or cancer of the uterus
- Hysterectomy for health problems that affect the uterus

What Is DES and Who Are Its Daughters?

Diethylstilbestrol (DES) is a synthetic form of the female hormone estrogen. Between 1940 and 1971, it was prescribed to pregnant women to prevent miscarriage, premature labor, and related complications of pregnancy. The use of DES declined after studies in the 1950s showed that it was not effective in preventing these problems.

In 1971, researchers linked prenatal (before birth) DES exposure to a type of cancer of the cervix and vagina (clear cell adenocarcinoma) in a small group of women. Soon after, the Food and Drug Administration (FDA) notified physicians throughout the country that DES should not be prescribed to pregnant women.

DES is now known to be an endocrine-disrupting chemical, one of a number of substances that interfere with the endocrine system to cause cancer, birth defects, and other developmental abnormalities. The effects of endocrine-disrupting chemicals are most severe when exposure occurs during fetal development.

For the daughters of women who used DES while pregnant—commonly called DES daughters—the risk of developing clear cell adenocarcinoma of the lower genital tract is approximately forty times higher than in unexposed women. However, this type of cancer is still rare. Generally speaking, only 1 in 1,000 DES daughters develop it.

The first DES daughters who were diagnosed with clear cell adenocarcinoma were very young at the time of their diagnoses. Subsequent research has shown that the risk of developing this disease remains elevated as women reach their forties.

DES daughters have an increased risk of developing abnormal cells in the cervix and the vagina that are precursors of cancer (dysplasia, cervical intraepithelial neoplasia, and squamous intraepithelial lesions). These abnormal cells resemble cancer cells, but they do not invade nearby healthy tissue and are *not* cancer. They may develop into cancer, however, if left untreated. It has been recommended that DES daughters have a yearly Pap test and pelvic exam to check for abnormal cells.

─────────── **MY JOURNEY** ───────────

During the fall of 2013, I began to experience discomfort in my "female region" and figured I just had some kind of infection, which would go away as they all had before, some naturally and the occasional one with a mild antibiotic. But even after I took a round of meds, something wasn't feeling quite right, and several months later I noticed a second bit of blood. (I had ignored the first one a few months earlier.)

I finally went to my doctor, who found what was deemed to be a common polyp on my vaginal wall. Even though vaginal cancer is rare, I went to see a special surgeon, who said the chance of it being cancerous was less than 5 percent. Well, even though I consider myself to be relatively average, it turned out I was quite unique because I was diagnosed with vaginal squamous cell cancer.

It was scary, but also really embarrassing, and while I didn't have trouble telling people I had cancer, I wasn't comfortable at all saying I had *vaginal* cancer! I just couldn't get over what it might have suggested. Silly, I know, but true nonetheless.

I found out that I had an even rarer form because cancers of the vagina usually occur when a cancer somewhere else spreads there. In my case, the cancer originated in the vagina, which probably explains why the doctor first thought it was a benign polyp. As an older woman, I mean one of retirement age, I learned that it was not so shocking to get this at my age.

Well, to make a long story short, after multiple rounds of radiation and a complicated surgical procedure, I was cancer-free.

Annabelle (Grand Rapids, Michigan)

Signs and Symptoms of Vaginal Cancer

The existence of vaginal cancer does not often cause early signs or symptoms. It may be found during a routine pelvic exam and Pap test. Signs and symptoms of vaginal cancer may include the following:

- Bleeding or discharge not related to menstrual periods
- Pain during sexual intercourse
- Pain in the pelvic area
- A lump in the vagina
- Pain when urinating
- Constipation

Tests that examine the vagina and other organs in the pelvis are used to detect and diagnose vaginal cancer. These include a thorough physical examination, including a family history (especially for possible exposure to DES), a pelvic exam, and Pap test.

Additional tests include the following:

- *Colposcopy:* A procedure in which a colposcope (a lighted, magnifying instrument) is used to check the vagina and cervix for abnormal areas. Tissue samples may be taken using a curette (spoon-shaped instrument) or a brush, which is then checked under a microscope for signs of disease.
- *Biopsy:* If abnormal cells are found in a Pap test, or a suspicious area is seen during a colposcopy, your doctor may do a biopsy. A sample of tissue is removed and viewed under a microscope by a pathologist to check for signs of cancer.

------------ MY JOURNEY ------------

As soon as I heard the doctor say *vagina* in the same sentence as *cancer*, my first thought had nothing to do with death or anything fatalistic like that. All I could think was, "My vagina? Are you kidding me? Can I still have sex?" I was happily married and sex was a healthy and very happy part of my life, so besides v-cancer, which was no doubt bad enough, having it in that specific place really sucked. It was even worse having to explain it to my husband and the rest of my family and friends.

Once my treatment started, I didn't think I could handle having that part of my life shut down, but, fortunately, it didn't last that long, and we have slowly but surely found our way back—not exactly to our former ways, but to an intimacy perhaps even richer.

Phyllis (Honolulu, Hawaii)

What Is VaIN? Can It Lead to Cancer?

VaIN is an acronym for vaginal intraepithelial neoplasia, which is just a technical description of the precise location of the disease and the cells it affects. VaIN is a rare, precancerous condition that *can* lead to cancer. The cause of VaIN and vaginal cancer is the same as the cause of cervical cancer—persistent infection with high-risk strains of HPV (Chapter 8). But vaginal cancer is about 100 times less common than cervical cancer for reasons having to do with biological differences between the two tissues.

The number of cases of vaginal cancer has been increasing, but this is primarily due to the increased frequency of doctors looking for it, using screening methods such as Pap smears and colposcopy. Early detection of VaIN can be difficult because patients usually lack symptoms.

VaIN analysis is based on how deep the abnormal cells are in the tissue lining the vagina. In VaIN 1, abnormal cells are found in the outermost one-third of the tissue lining the vagina. In VaIN 2, abnormal cells are found in the outermost two-thirds of the tissue lining the vagina. In VaIN 3, abnormal cells are found in more than two-thirds of the tissue lining the vagina. When abnormal cells are found throughout the tissue lining, it is called carcinoma *in situ.*

Defining Terms

Epithelium: This is just the outer layer of cells that line the surfaces of the vagina and vulva. The term *intraepithelial* simply means that the disease is in this layer of cells and hasn't spread beyond it.

Neoplasia: This literally means "new growth" and refers to an abnormal growth of tissue and is used to refer to both cancer and precancerous conditions.

You can see that the condition called *v*aginal *i*ntraepithelial *neo*plasia (VaIN) can be translated as a new, abnormal growth of tissue in the outer layer of cells that line the vagina.

Treatment of VaIN and Vaginal Cancer

The goal of treating VaIN and vaginal cancer is to relieve any symptoms, prevent the development of invasive cancer, and avoid surgeries that may be disfiguring and interfere with sexual function.

Topical therapy is the application of the prescribed drug, dissolved in a cream, directly in contact with the cancer or precancer, instead of swallowing it in a pill or receiving it through an injection. This method is used to treat vaginal precancer (VaIN) but is not used to treat invasive vaginal cancer.

One such drug is called *imiquimod* (Aldara or Zyclara). This drug is approved by the FDA for treating genital warts caused by HPV, but many doctors use the drug "off label" to treat other HPV-caused diseases, such as VaIN and VIN. Imiquimod works by triggering the body's immune system of natural killer cells to attack and eliminate the abnormal or cancerous cells.

Because of its effect on the immune system, imiquimod may cause side effects, such as redness, swelling, or burning in the area where the cream is applied. Patients can also experience flu-like symptoms.

Fluorouracil (5-FU) is a chemotherapy drug, typically given intravenously. However, it can also be applied directly to the lining of the vagina. This is repeated either once a week for ten weeks or applied each night for one to two weeks. The main drawback is that it can cause severe irritation in the vaginal and vulvar area. In addition, it may not be as effective as using a laser or simply removing the lesion with surgery.

Another nonsurgical treatment of VaIN and VIN is called photodynamic therapy. Special drugs called photosensitizing agents are usually painted on the area containing the precancer and then—after the abnormal cells have absorbed the drug—a special light is shined on the area. This light activates the drug, which then kills the cells.

Early stage tumors are often curable with local modality therapies, but there is no standard treatment of proven efficacy for metastatic disease. A large proportion (30 to 50 percent) of women with vaginal carcinomas have had a prior hysterectomy for benign, premalignant, or malignant disease.

Surgery is the most common treatment of cancer that has already invaded the deeper tissues. The following surgical procedures may be used:

- Laser surgery uses a narrow beam of intense light as a knife to make bloodless cuts in tissue or to remove a surface lesion such as a tumor.
- Wide local excision removes the cancer and some of the healthy tissue around it.
- Vaginectomy removes all or part of the vagina.
- Total hysterectomy removes the uterus, including the cervix.

Skin grafting may follow surgery in order to repair or reconstruct the vagina. This is a surgical procedure in which skin is moved from one part of the body to another. A piece of healthy skin is taken from a part of the body that is usually hidden, such as the buttock or thigh, and used to repair or rebuild the area treated with surgery.

Even if the doctor removes all the cancer that can be seen during surgery, some patients may be given radiation therapy after surgery to kill any microscopic cancer cells that are left.

———————— MY JOURNEY ————————

When I first heard the expression referring to "getting hit below the belt," it pertained to my little brother, who, while swinging at a pitch during his first Little League game, missed the ball, which quickly hit him you know where—below the belt. But he was only nine years old, and the ball wasn't coming in too fast, so he gasped for a second and got over it with an embarrassed smile. We laughed and hoped he would recover with a monster home run. He ended up drawing a walk, which wasn't such a bad alternative for him or his team.

Many years later, when I was diagnosed with cancer of the vagina, I reminded him of that game when I told him, "Henry, I just got hit below the belt with a very unexpected pitch." We sort of laughed until we didn't, and once we stopped crying we started hoping that I would recover with a home run, or something close, at least. I actually was happy to settle for a walk, as in walking out of the hospital after surgery and continuing to walk each and every day until the cancer was gone.

Lucky for me, I found amazing teammates among the many women I met facing similar circumstances. Discovering I was not alone played a huge role in my recovery, and that happened only when I was willing to come out of my own closet, leaving the self-pity behind to face a new pitcher on the mound—my own life—with whatever adjustments I had to make in my batting stance. Sorry for all the baseball metaphors, but they apply, and it's good to go to a game every now and then and remember that I *am* part of a community.

Susan (Wilmington, Delaware)

VIN: Two Precancerous Conditions May Lead to Two Types of Vulvar Cancer

VIN stands for vulvar intraepithelial neoplasia and is a precancerous condition. VIN consists of patches of abnormal cells on the surface of the vulva. Based on biopsies of tissues, pathologists diagnose two distinct types of VIN.

1. *uVIN* (usual VIN) is more common, affects women beginning in their forties, and is caused by persistent infection with HPV. About 6 percent of uVINs progress to cancer.
2. *dVIN* (differentiated VIN) is less common and affects women in their sixties after menopause. dVIN arises out of certain chronic inflammatory diseases of the vulva, including lichen sclerosis. About one-third of dVINs progress to cancer.

Skin Conditions

Lichen sclerosis is a chronic inflammation of the skin that most often affects the anus and genital regions, including the vulva. Its symptoms include pain, intense itching, and painful intercourse. Lichen sclerosis can occur at any age but is most common in two age groups: young girls before puberty and women after menopause.

It can be difficult for non-dermatologists to diagnose correctly. The cause of lichen sclerosis is unknown, but it may be an autoimmune disease for which patients have a genetic predisposition. There is no cure for lichen sclerosis, but it is effectively treated with prescription steroid creams.

Diagnosis of VIN and Vulvar Cancers

About 60 percent of women with VIN experience itching and pain, and their gynecologist may see pale-whitish patches or raised areas or pimples that merge or grow together.

Vulvar cancer, which most often affects the outer vaginal lips, does not usually cause early signs or symptoms but may cause any of the following:

- A lump or growth on the vulva
- Changes in the vulvar skin, such as color changes or growths that look like a wart or ulcer
- Itching in the vulvar area that does not go away
- Tenderness or pain in the vulvar area
- Bleeding

Vulvar cancer usually forms slowly. In VIN, abnormal cells can grow on the surface of the vulvar skin over a long period of time. Because it is possible for VIN to become vulvar cancer, it is very important to get treatment. For suspected VINs and vulvar cancers, your gynecologist will do a biopsy and submit it to the clinical laboratory for diagnosis by a pathologist.

——————————— MY JOURNEY ———————————

Since being diagnosed with vulvar cancer almost seven years ago,
I have made a constant effort to find other women in the same boat.

Since my surgery, when my doctor told me I probably had just a few more good years left, I have volleyed back and forth on a fairly steady basis between misery and despair, elation and relief. For better or worse, this roller-coaster ride, which doesn't recognize logic or available science, has been my main mode of transportation for *more* than "a few" years. I am happy to report, and with my newfound thirst for knowledge about everything related to my body and soul, I plan on extending that for several more, at the very least. By the way, I found a new surgeon, had two more surgeries, and finally feel confident in sharing my story.

Lorraine (Sacramento, California)

Risk Factors for Vulvar Cancer

Risk factors for vulvar cancer include the following:

- Having vulvar intraepithelial neoplasia (VIN)
- Having human papillomavirus (HPV) infection
  (See Chapter 8 for more information about HPV infection)
- History of genital warts

Other possible risk factors include the following:

- Multiple sexual partners
- First sexual intercourse at a young age
- History of abnormal Pap tests (Pap smears)

Treatment of VINs and Vulvar Cancers

The goals of treatment and treatment of VINs are similar to those of VaINs. Vulvar cancers can be treated using different surgical procedures depending on how far and deep the tumor has spread. The goals of these procedures are to remove all of the cancer while preserving the patient's sexual functions if possible. They include the following:

- *Laser surgery:* An intense, focused beam of light vaporizes the layers of skin containing the abnormal cells.
- *Wide local excision:* This is performed if large areas of skin need to be removed. Skin grafts from other parts of the body may be used to cover the wound.
- *Skinning vulvectomy:* A procedure where only the top layer of skin affected by the cancer is removed.
- *Simple vulvectomy:* This procedure removes not only the skin but also some of the underlying tissue.
- *Radical vulvectomy:* This removes the entire vulva and local lymph nodes.

Even if all of the cancer that can be seen at the time of the surgery is removed, some patients may have chemotherapy or radiation therapy after surgery to kill any remaining cancer cells. Treatment given after the surgery to lower the risk that the cancer will come back is called adjuvant therapy.

KEY POINTS TO REMEMBER

✓ Cancers of the vagina and vulva are much less common than other gynecologic cancers.

✓ Most cancers of the vagina and vulva are caused by HPV and can be prevented by HPV vaccines (Chapter 8).

✓ For the daughters of women who used DES (diethylstil-bestrol) while pregnant, the risk of developing cancer of the lower genital tract is approximately forty times higher than in unexposed women.

✓ Vulvar and vaginal cancers do not often cause early signs or symptoms.

✓ Vulvar cancer usually forms slowly over several years.

✓ The development of vulvar cancers is preceded by precancerous conditions that, if caught early, can be cured by surgery.

✓ The goal of treatment is to do just enough to get rid of the cancer and, at the same time, preserve the patient's sexual functioning.

TRACE OF LIGHT

Deep beneath
The weight of knowing
Cancer's grip
On Weeks, months,
Years.

A trace of light
Breaks through.
Shrouded still,
Stained
With fear.

The prescription simple:
Live while you are here,
What grows inside
Provides only
A suggested passage.

Shelter
Beckons.
Light is there.
Travelers
Arriving Daily.

—Ellen McGaughey

10 WHAT AM I DEALING WITH? Defining Short-Term Challenges of Treatment

My cancer scare changed my life.
I'm grateful for every new, healthy day I have.
It has helped me prioritize my life.

—Olivia Newton-John

Do Your Due Diligence

Any cancer treatment can cause challenging side effects. Problems may arise when treatment designed to impact cancerous tissues also affects healthy tissues or organs. Each person undergoing a treatment regimen reacts to it in his or her individual way. Some people experience very few side effects while others may need to endure more than they anticipated.

Several factors contribute to the side effects you may experience, including the type of treatment, its amount or frequency, your age, and any other health conditions you may already have. Most of the short-term side effects discussed in this chapter will improve after treatment has ended, although some may take weeks or months to resolve completely.

> **NOTE to PATIENT:**
> Before you begin any kind of treatment,
> ask your healthcare team which side effects are
> likely to present challenges. Learn about the steps you
> can take to lessen them, during—and after—treatment.

Surgery: What Are the General Risks and Side Effects?

Complications during surgery can be caused by the procedure itself; the drugs used before, during, and/or after the procedure (including the anesthesia); or any underlying disease a patient may already have. In general, the more complex the surgery the greater the risk.

Surgical procedures today are generally safer than they have ever been. Technical advances, including less invasive, microsurgical and robotic surgical techniques have improved safety levels and shortened recovery time. Despite these breakthroughs, there is always a small risk to any surgical procedure. Some of these include the following:

- Bleeding
- Damage to nearby tissues, such as blood vessels or nerves
- Reactions to drugs or anesthesia used during the procedure
- Damage to other organs, such as the lungs, heart, or kidneys (more common if you already have conditions that affect these organs)

———————————— MY JOURNEY ————————————

I was self-conscious immediately after my surgery because of the large scar on my chest. If anyone other than my doctor or a nurse saw it, I freaked out. I didn't even want my husband—and, God forbid, my kids—to see it. But gradually I convinced myself that I was going to be me, no matter what I looked like. When someone at the beach told me I looked beautiful—in my humongous one-piece—I was embarrassed but thrilled. It showed me that I must be making progress from the inside out, not just from the outside in. In a matter of weeks, I was back to wearing a two-piece suit and feeling comfortable in my own skin.

Ronda (Sarasota, Florida)

The most common post-operative problems after surgery include the following:

- *Pain:* This is normal after any surgery and its frequency and level depends on how extensive a procedure you have had, as well as your individual pain threshold. Medications for pain relief range from acetaminophen to stronger drugs, such as codeine and morphine. Some of them are dispensed in pill form, while others may be included in a post-op IV.
- *Infections:* The most likely location is at the surgical site. Your doctor may prescribe antibiotics prophylactically or later if there are any signs of infection. They may be given by mouth or through a vein. Contracting pneumonia is possible for any patient with previously impaired lung function, such as smokers, or if pain from the procedure prevents the patient from taking deep breaths.
- *Slow recovery of other body functions:* Symptoms such as

decreased bowel activity may occur after surgery due to inactivity, change in diet, and medications.

Sandra Lee: Cancer-Free at Last

In March 2015, Food Network celebrity chef Sandra Lee was diagnosed with early breast cancer, specifically ductal carcinoma *in situ* (DCIS). Six months later, her doctors told her she was cancer-free. But her path was not easy. In August of that year, the forty-nine-year-old *Semi-Homemade Cooking* host was rushed to the hospital when she experienced "an extremely painful fluid buildup" in the area where she had undergone a bilateral mastectomy in May.

An infection had developed at the mastectomy site, so Lee had another surgical procedure to clear it out. She also required two weeks of intravenous antibiotics administered through a mediport, a small, plastic disc that is inserted under the skin, which is used to reduce the need for inserting an intravenous (IV) line each time treatment is required. A soft, thin tube, called a catheter, is inserted from the port into a large vein. In many cases, a special needle with medication can be attached to the port.

Six months after her initial diagnosis, and following the additional treatment of the infection, Sandra Lee's doctors declared her cancer-free.

How to Recognize an Infection

Any type of cancer treatment can cause complications, including an infection, which is an invasion and growth of germs in the body, such as bacteria, viruses, yeast, or other fungi. An infection can begin anywhere. It may spread throughout the body and can cause one or more of these signs:

- Fever of 100.5°F (38°C) or higher or chills
- Cough or sore throat
- Diarrhea
- Ear pain, headache or sinus pain, or a stiff or sore neck
- Skin rash
- Sores or white coating in the mouth or on the tongue
- Swelling or redness, especially where a catheter enters the body
- Urine that is bloody or cloudy, or pain when urinating

> **NOTE to PATIENT:**
> Call your healthcare team if you have signs of an infection.
> Infections during cancer treatment can be life threatening
> and require urgent medical attention.

Radiation Therapy: General Risks and Side Effects

Radiation therapy destroys cancer cells by damaging their DNA (the molecules inside cells that carry genetic information and pass it from one generation to the next). It can either damage DNA directly or create charged particles (free radicals) within the cells that, in turn, can damage the DNA. Cancer cells containing DNA that is damaged beyond repair will stop dividing and self-destruct. When the damaged cells die, they are broken down and eliminated naturally by the body.

Unfortunately, radiation therapy can also damage normal cells, leading to side effects. Doctors take this into account when planning a course of therapy. The amount of radiation that normal tissue can safely receive is known for all parts of the body. Doctors use this information to help them decide where to aim radiation most effectively.

Radiation therapy can cause both early (acute) and late (chronic) side effects. Acute side effects occur during treatment, and chronic side

effects occur months or even years after treatment ends. The type of
side effect depends on the area of the body being treated, the daily dose
of radiation, as well as the total dose received, your general medical
health, and other treatments you may be receiving at the same time.

Acute radiation side effects are caused by damage to rapidly dividing normal cells in the area of treatment. These effects can include skin
irritation, dry mouth, hair loss, or urinary problems, again depending
upon the area of the body being treated. Most acute effects disappear
after treatment ends, though some can be permanent.

Fatigue is a common side effect of radiation therapy, regardless of
which part of the body is treated. Nausea with or without vomiting
is common when the abdomen is treated and occurs sometimes with
treatment of the brain. Medications are available to help prevent or
treat nausea and vomiting during treatment.

There are two main types of radiation therapy.

1. *External beam radiation:* This therapy comes from a machine
   that aims radiation at your cancer. The machine is large and
   may be noisy. It does not touch you but can move around you,
   sending radiation to a part of your body from many directions. External beam radiation therapy treats a specific part of
   your body. For example, if you have cancer in your breast, you
   will have radiation only to your chest, not to your whole body.
2. *Internal radiation:* This therapy is distinguished by having a
   source of radiation put inside your body. The radiation source
   can be solid or liquid. Internal radiation therapy with a solid
   source is called brachytherapy. In this type of treatment,
   radiation in the form of seeds, ribbons, or capsules is placed in
   your body in or near the cancer. You receive liquid radiation
   through an IV line, which allows the liquid to travel throughout your body, seeking out and killing cancer cells.

MY JOURNEY

No matter what, I refuse to be robbed of my sexuality. Forget about losing hair, running to the bathroom, or falling asleep in the middle of my favorite movie. I make love to my husband like always, which helps me feel like myself—alive! I forget everything I'm afraid of when we are together like that, and if and when I start to cry or get upset at the wrong moment, we just have to laugh, because what else is there to do?

Marie (Garden City, New York)

Chemotherapy: General Risks and Side Effects

Like radiation therapy, chemotherapy works by stopping or slowing the growth of cancer cells, which grow and divide quickly. But it can also harm healthy cells, which divide quickly, including cells in your skin, hair, nails, the lining of your digestive system, and your blood cells.

Damage to healthy cells is the cause of side effects. Most side effects lessen or go away after chemotherapy has ended. Common short-term side effects of chemotherapy include the following:

- *Hair loss:* Although it may be most notable when the hair on your head falls out, hair loss from chemotherapy can occur all over the body, including the eyelashes and eyebrows.
- *Nausea and vomiting:* Antinausea drugs are often given to mitigate these side effects.
- *Nail weakness:* The nails may become brittle, break easily, or develop ridges in them.
- *Pain:* Some chemotherapy can cause temporary nerve damage, which presents itself as burning or shooting pain. The specific

symptoms will depend on which peripheral nerves (sensory, motor, or autonomic) are affected.

- *Muscle soreness:* This can also be caused by chemotherapy and will usually go away after treatment is stopped, but it may take several weeks or months to resolve.
- *Mouth pain and sore throat* (mucositis/stomatitis): Chemotherapy causes irritation of the lining of the mouth and throat, making it difficult to eat and swallow.
- *Fatigue/tiredness:* This can happen randomly and not always corresponding with treatment.
- *Constipation/diarrhea:* It may be isolated or may become chronic.
- *Loss of menstruation or menopausal symptoms:* If this occurs during treatment, consult with the appropriate doctor.
- *Anemia:* This refers to a low red blood cell count. It can be manifested as fatigue, shortness of breath, and paleness.
- *Leukopenia and neutropenia:* Both refer to a low white blood cell count. It can increase your risk of infection or make you subject to infections that healthy people don't normally get.
- *Increased bruising:* This is usually due to low platelet counts.

―――――――――――― **MY JOURNEY** ――――――――――――

From my experience, one of the best upsides of losing your hair during chemotherapy is the chance to obtain a whole new look—new length, style, and new color, or any combination. That's because a good wig store represents unlimited possibilities. I found an amazing place to get what soon became a collection, because I found out quite early that one wig would simply not be enough. If cancer was going to mess me up, I was determined to make the most of it, and I decided that I could start feeling better if I took care of my hair.

The wig store had them on display in all their glory, and I quickly became a kid in a candy store. I mean, I was picking one for wearing around the house, one for shopping, one to go to my kids' school, and another for those rare nights when my husband and I went out alone. Of course, I had to have a really special one for special occasions, like going shopping for another wig!

The store even had names for them, but I often changed them once I got home. My favorite name for my "everyday" wig became "Blessing," which I thought was ironic but somehow true. Cancer is a terrible thing, but it can also be a blessing, especially for those of us who are able to learn so much about ourselves throughout the whole process. So wherever I went, Blessing was with me, protecting my head—not only from the elements but from my own head exploding with insecurity.

Look, it sucked losing my hair. Not just the hair on my head, either. But look at it this way. I didn't have to comb it for several months, and once it grew back, I was well equipped with a little boutique of my own, ready for many years of trick or treating. What a blessing.

Fatima (Austin, Texas)

Symptoms of Peripheral Neuropathy

Neuropathy refers to nerve disease or damage. Peripheral nerves send signals to the brain through the spinal cord, such as "my feet are cold" or "stand up." Any damage to this communication system may cause a person to experience compromised movement and feeling.

According to the National Institute of Neurological Disorders and Stroke (part of the NIH), approximately 20 million people in the United States experience some form of peripheral neuropathy, a condition that develops as a result of damage to the peripheral nervous system, which can be triggered by certain cancer treatments.

Damage to sensory nerves—those that help you feel pain, heat, cold, and pressure—may cause a variety of side effects, including tingling, numbness, or a pins-and-needles feeling in your feet and hands that may spread to your legs and arms, an inability to feel hot or cold sensations, or an inability to feel pain, such as from a cut or sore on your foot.

Damage to motor nerves—those that help your muscles move—can cause weak or achy muscles, which may cause you to lose your balance or trip easily. It may also be difficult to button shirts or open jars. This side effect may also make muscles twitch/cramp, and if you don't use your muscles regularly, it can cause what is called muscle wasting. If your chest or throat muscles are affected, this can become especially serious if it creates difficulties in swallowing or breathing.

Damage to autonomic nerves—those that control functions such as blood pressure, digestion, heart rate, temperature, and urination—can cause digestive changes, such as constipation or diarrhea, dizzy or faintness (due to low blood pressure), sexual problems (men may be unable to get an erection and women may not reach orgasm), sweating problems (either too much or too little), and/or urination problems, such as leaking urine or difficulty emptying your bladder.

> **NOTE to PATIENT:**
> If any of these side effects appear, inform your doctor!
> Don't wait until they become unmanageable.
> There are no stupid questions!

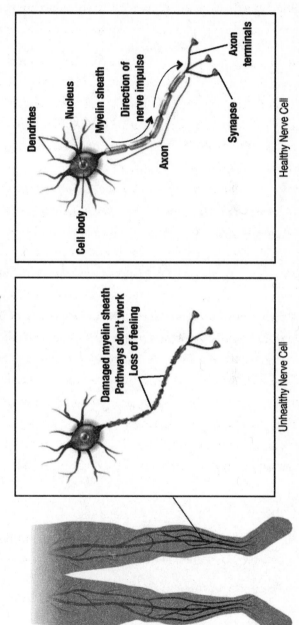

Peripheral Neuropathy
Nerve Damage

Dendrites
Nucleus
Myelin sheath
Direction of nerve impulse
Axon terminals
Cell body
Axon
Synapse

Healthy Nerve Cell

Damaged myelin sheath
Pathways don't work
Loss of feeling

Unhealthy Nerve Cell

Source: © Guniita (*Dreamstime.com*)

KEY POINTS TO REMEMBER

✓ Any kind of cancer treatment can cause challenging
   side effects.

✓ Most short-term side effects improve after treatment
   has ended, although some may take weeks or months
   to resolve completely.

✓ Before you begin any kind of treatment, ask your
   healthcare team which side effects are likely to present challenges. Learn about what you can do to lessen
   them, during—and after—treatment.

✓ Surgical procedures today are generally safer than they
   have ever been.

✓ Any type of cancer treatment can cause complications,
   including an infection, which is an invasion and growth
   of germs in the body, such as bacteria, viruses, yeast,
   or other fungi.

✓ Call your healthcare team if you have signs of an
   infection. They can become life threatening and require
   urgent medical attention.

✓ Fatigue is a common side effect of radiation therapy.

✓ Neuropathy refers to nerve disease or damage.

✓ If side effects appear, inform your doctor! Don't wait
   until they become unmanageable.

✓ There are no stupid questions!

I'm Becoming More Forgetful

I am becoming more forgetful.
Friends laugh
tell stories about
misplaced keys
forgotten names.
A few gently ask if chemo did this to me.
My doctor refers me for an MRI.
You don't understand.
For just one moment
I forgot that I
have/had/may have
cancer.

I have become a magician
watching in amazement
as fear disappears.
Sounds of audible delight escape
as the faint outline
of hope
materializes,
and as hope takes shape
remembering begins.

—Jane Levin

11

WHO HAVE I BECOME? Defining Long-Term Challenges of Cancer Survivorship

Having cancer does make you try to be better at
everything you do and enjoy every moment.
It changes you forever.
But it can be a positive change.

—Jaclyn Smith, as told to *Coping* magazine

What Does It Mean to Be a Survivor?

You've finished your treatments and have been given the "all clear" from your doctor. But for many cancer patients, you may experience lingering, or even new side effects apart from the surgical scars. This chapter discusses some of the long-term complications and risks after treatment.

For example, Olympic gold medalist Dorothy Hamill is still coping with fatigue years after her breast cancer treatment. *Fashion Police*'s Guiliana Rancic has been struggling with the effects of dramatic weight loss, a side effect caused by a medication she has been on since her double mastectomy four years ago. Reality personality Diem Brown tried to preserve her fertility despite an ovarian cancer diagnosis. And *Good Morning America* anchor Robin Roberts's battle with myelodysplastic syndrome (MDS) demonstrates how cancer treatment can cause a second cancer, years after the first has been cured.

So what does it really mean to be a survivor?

Most people define it as someone who has overcome something, who has reached the other side of what may be the most difficult journey of their lives. Each individual will see the process differently and will vary on how they identify with the word itself, especially when determining when they become a survivor and how long that status applies. Since we can't foresee the future, and the concept of survivorship is not an exact science, we can only suggest that each patient approach these long-term challenges one day at a time.

Since this chapter explores an assortment of long-term effects—physical, psychological, and emotional—of cancer treatments, let's begin at the top, with "mission control."

Chemo Brain: When Thoughts and Feelings Run Amok

According to the National Cancer Institute, one in four people with cancer report memory and attention problems after chemotherapy. Doctors call this phenomenon chemotherapy-related cognitive dysfunction, which is commonly referred to as chemo brain.

Many survivors describe it as a "brain fog," which can lead to problems with paying attention, trouble finding the right words, difficulty remembering new things, trouble multitasking, memory lapses, and taking longer to do things due to disorganized, slower thinking and mental processing.

These effects can begin soon after treatment ends, or they may not appear until much later. They don't always go away. If a person is older, it can be hard to tell whether these changes in memory and concentration are a result of treatment or of the aging process. Either way, some feel they just can't focus as they once did.

Research is starting to explore why some people develop problems with memory and concentration while others don't. It seems that people who have had chemotherapy or have had radiation to the head area are at higher risk for these problems. People who had high doses of chemotherapy may have memory problems, but even those who had standard doses have reported memory changes.

Although chemo brain was first identified and named by breast cancer survivors, research now suggests that the same constellation of symptoms also affects survivors of other cancers.

It may not be only the cancer treatment that causes chemo brain. Dr. Tim Ahles, who studies chemo brain at Memorial Sloan-Kettering Cancer Center in New York City, explains that some patients tested before starting treatment may have cognitive problems. He suggests, "Aspects of cancer biology may influence cognitive functioning, or that there are as-yet-unidentified shared risk factors for mild cognitive changes and the development of cancer. It's more complicated than chemotherapy. Almost no one who is treated for cancer receives only chemotherapy. Other aspects of treatment may be equally important to understanding changes in cognitive functioning."[17]

Studies have been done using something called functional magnetic resonance imaging (fMRI), a technology that measures brain activity

---

17. *http://www.cancer.gov/about-cancer/treatment/research/understanding-chemobrain*

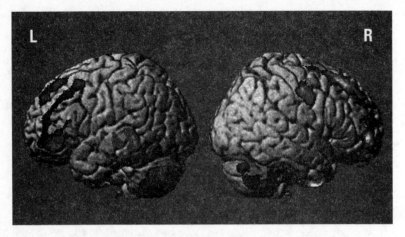

*Chemo Brain. An MRI scan shows decreases in gray matter in
the brain's bilateral frontal lobes and cerebellum and right
temporal lobe after one month of chemotherapy.*
Source: Brenna C. McDonald (used with permission)

by detecting changes associated with blood flow. This technique relies
on the fact that cerebral blood flow and neuronal activation are cou-
pled. When an area of the brain is in use, blood flow to that region
also increases. Using this method, researchers have identified structural
brain abnormalities in patients treated with chemotherapy.

In another study, this time using positron emission tomography
(PET) imaging, breast cancer survivors who had received chemotherapy during the previous five to ten years used more of their brains to
perform a short-term memory task than control subjects who had
never received chemotherapy—a sign that their brains are having to
work harder to complete the task.

Dr. Ahles, along with colleagues at Dartmouth Medical School,
suggest that a form, or allele, of the APOE gene, called ε4, may be
a genetic marker for increased vulnerability to chemo brain. This
marker is also associated with increased risk for Alzheimer's disease.

They looked at a large number of long-term breast and lymphoma survivors and found that participants who had at least one ε4 allele had significantly lower scores on standard tests of visual memory and spatial ability and a tendency toward lower scores on psychomotor functioning than subjects who did not carry this allele.

Dr. Patricia Ganz and her colleagues at UCLA's Jonsson Comprehensive Cancer Center suspect that uncontrolled inflammation may be a cause of chemo brain. "Many of the patients in our breast cancer survivorship program who have cognitive complaints also have fatigue, sleep disturbance, or depression," she said. "Our hypothesis is that small differences [called polymorphisms] in genes that regulate the immune system render some patients more vulnerable to this constellation of symptoms."

Many cancer treatments, including surgery, radiation, chemotherapy, and immunotherapy, can increase inflammation, Dr. Ganz added, which may not resolve after treatment ends.

Research on treatments for chemo brain is still in its very early stages. Dr. Ganz is beginning a pilot study of rehabilitation strategies for affected breast cancer survivors. Some evidence suggests that medications that stimulate the central nervous system, such as Adderall (dextroamphetamine-amphetamine), may moderate adverse cognitive effects.

Amy Robach: Inspiring Others While Saving Herself

On October 1, 2011, as part of Breast Cancer Awareness Month, *Good Morning America (GMA)* news correspondent Amy Robach agreed to do an onscreen mammogram (her first) to promote cancer screening. At forty years old (the age when screening routinely starts), Robach had been putting off the test and was initially reluctant to do it in front of millions of viewers. But *GMA* producers and coworker and breast cancer survivor Robin Roberts convinced her that getting the mammogram on air could potentially save the life of a woman who decides to get her own mammogram because of watching Robach. Little did she know that she was about to save her own life.

Just a few hours after undergoing her onscreen mammogram as part of the promotional event, Amy was called back to the clinic for what she thought were just "a few follow-up images." But she received the news that she had breast cancer. She underwent a bilateral mastectomy followed by eight rounds of chemotherapy. Astonishingly, Robach remained on the air throughout the process, taking only a week off for reconstructive surgery.

In June 2014, during an in-depth interview with the *New York Daily News*,[18] Robach revealed some of the side effects she experienced due to the chemotherapy, especially with her memory. "The chemo brain, the chemo fog, is a real thing. I would have conversations with people, they would take pictures with me after the show, and they would send them to me and say thank you . . . it took my breath away—it upset me tremendously because I actually wouldn't be able to remember taking that picture or having a conversation, and for me that was one of the hardest side effects of chemo. I was so afraid I was gonna drop the ball or just do or say something stupid because I wasn't in my sharpest mode."

Emotional Distress and Depression

For some, dealing with cancer can lead to serious depression and emotional distress. These feelings may be strongest during the first year after diagnosis, and they can manifest themselves in a variety of physical ways.

---

18. *http://www.nydailynews.com/entertainment/tv/amy-robach-good-morning-america-details-breast-cancer-battle-article-1.1839892*

One of the most common residual effects of any cancer experience is a fear of recurrence. After cancer treatment ends, many people are afraid that they still have cancer or that it will come back. These fears are normal. For some people, talking to a counselor or joining a support group can be helpful. Your healthcare provider may be able to help you find a counselor or support group. Others may choose to seek other therapeutic options, including art therapy, expressive writing classes or journal clubs, or joining a theater group of survivors.

Volunteering at the cancer center where you were treated may also be helpful. There's nothing more hopeful for a patient in the midst of a difficult treatment protocol than to see someone else who is surviving and thriving after going through the same thing. And providing that optimism may also offer you the positive boost you may need from time to time.

Insomnia

Whether it's anxiety, lack of quality sleep, or fluctuations in diet and exercise, any of us can experience challenges in getting adequate sleep, which can occur from the normal stressors of everyday life.

But a diagnosis of cancer can easily compound these normal tendencies, and it can easily lead to insomnia if we are not careful. This can be especially troublesome because when cancer is present, our bodies naturally become more sensitive and vulnerable, and it becomes increasingly important that we get adequate sleep not only to heal physically but to give our minds and hearts the chance to enjoy a quality rest.

Medications are often used to treat insomnia in people without cancer, yet only a few studies show that they reduce insomnia specifically related to cancer treatment.

Here are some other things you can do to get a better night's sleep:

- Keep a regular schedule and avoid napping during the day.
- Avoid spicy foods, caffeine, and alcohol before bedtime.
- Sleep in a dark, quiet place.
- Reduce tension with meditation or other relaxation techniques.
- Keep your bedroom as screen-free as possible, that includes televisions, laptops, smartphones, etc.

Hormones and Fertility

Everyone's natural hormone levels change during their lifetime, but women, due to events like puberty, pregnancy, and menopause, are susceptible to a special type of roller coaster ride. Continuing research in the intersection of cancer and endocrinology—the study of the endocrine system, which includes our hormones and the glands that produce them—reveals how our chosen lifestyles, including consumption of alcohol and food, can affect hormone levels and the risk of getting cancer. This also applies to hormonal medicines, such as birth-control pills, menopausal hormone therapy (HT or MHT), and hormone replacement therapy (HRT).

Menopausal hormone therapy, in particular, has been used for decades to manage symptoms of menopause, and doctors and patients swore by their health benefits, but, according to the American Cancer Society, studies have led many doctors to conclude that the risks may often outweigh the benefits and can affect a woman's risk of getting certain cancers.

Regarding fertility and cancer, most women, whether they end up having children or not, at least want to preserve the option. Cancer—and its subsequent treatments—may compromise or even eliminate this possibility. For many women, pursuing a pregnancy or preserving the chance to later can become a complicated and excruciating decision.

Understanding any or all of these factors will help you navigate this difficult road.

Seeking advice *before* treatment is crucial.

Early Menopause

This can occur in any woman undergoing cancer treatment, even in those who have not had their ovaries removed. Chemotherapy and/ or radiation therapy can have damaging effects on the ovaries and can stop your menstrual cycle. In women younger than forty years of age, the effect is usually temporary. However, for women over forty it may be permanent.

In either situation, menopause can trigger significant emotional responses beyond any physical symptoms, which include hot flashes, night sweats, and vaginal dryness. Because of the sudden nature of menopause caused by chemo and/or radiation therapy, symptoms may be more severe. Unless you are treated with hormone replacement therapy (HRT), early menopause can affect the health of your bones, leading to osteoporosis, a condition that causes bones to become weak and brittle.

--- **MY JOURNEY** ---

Under ideal circumstances, a woman will face menopause with gently open arms when her body is naturally ready. But since life has a habit of being naughty, many women, including me, have had to face this change prematurely, and this creates havoc, not just for the body, but for the soul. As I was getting older, well before I got cancer, several women told me that menopause was something to welcome, that it would make me more mellow and wise, leading to a confidence I probably never felt before. Well, I love those women, but they were wrong. When I was smacked upside down with menopause as a result of my cancer treatment, I was enraged, constantly agitated and totally resistant to my body being prematurely robbed of its still-emerging womanhood. I was thirty-five, for goodness sake! Now, after a year adapting to my new body and drastic changes in energy, I am trying to regain what motivates me each day to live. So far, I don't know if I will ever regain my sense of self. The challenge is to redefine what it takes to be me, and to do whatever it takes to get there. And since life is short, I'd better get busy!

—*Dalia (Memphis, Tennessee)*

Fertility Issues

More than 150,000 American women are diagnosed each year with cancer during their reproductive years (younger than age forty-five). Treatment for women's cancers can lead to infertility in a variety of ways. Surgical removal of the uterus, ovaries, cervix, and/or the vagina will interfere with the normal process of conception, pregnancy, and childbirth. And, as we previously mentioned, both chemotherapy and radiation therapy can lead to ovarian failure, and radiation therapy can lead to scarring in the pelvic region.

But modern technology has allowed many women to preserve their fertility.

If becoming a parent is important to you, talk with your physician *before* beginning any treatment. In 2006, the American Society of Clinical Oncology (ASCO) published guidelines recommending that oncologists discuss with all patients of reproductive age the possibility of treatment-related infertility, as well as options for preserving fertility, and provide them with referrals to reproductive specialists.

Diem Brown: One Challenge Too Many

As a contestant on MTV's *Real World/Road Rules Challenge* in 2006, Diem Brown expected to undergo a difficult journey. But the twenty-three-year-old did not expect the challenge one month after having surgery for ovarian cancer. Brown had one ovary, several lymph nodes, and part of her fallopian tube removed, but she still flew off to Australia to participate in the show. She and her partner, Derrick, finished in fourth place in the competition.

After successful treatment, Brown went on to be a cast member in MTV's *The Challenge* series, "The Duel" and "The Ruins." In May 2012, after experiencing abdominal pain, tests revealed that Diem had a large cyst in her remaining ovary. Her cancer had returned, and she underwent another surgery. Since the doctor was able to keep 30 percent of her remaining ovary when the cyst was removed, Brown decided to postpone treatment temporarily so that eggs could be harvested before the remainder of her ovary was removed as part of her treatment. In July 2012, Diem went to New York University, where she was able to have five eggs harvested.

Unfortunately, Diem was never able to use those eggs. In August 2014, her ovarian cancer returned, this time with multiple tumors in her colon, stomach, liver, and lymph nodes. Doctors removed part of her colon as well as her uterus. Despite her difficult situation, she remained upbeat and chronicled her cancer journey in a blog for *People* magazine. She passed away in November 2014 at the age of thirty-four.

Fertility Preservation Methods for Women

The two most common ways women can preserve their fertility before cancer treatments are egg and embryo freezing.

Egg freezing is the process of removing eggs from the ovaries and preserving them for future use. This may be an option prior to cancer treatment if you do not have a male partner, do not want to use donor sperm, or do not want to pursue embryo freezing at this time.

It consists of three main steps:

1. *Ovarian stimulation:* This involves the use of ovulation, or fertility drugs. These hormones, taken over a period of eight to fourteen days, stimulate a woman's ovaries to produce several eggs instead of one per menstrual cycle.

2. *Egg retrieval:* Once the eggs are deemed ready for retrieval, the doctor performs a transvaginal ultrasound aspiration. This is a simple surgical procedure that uses a small amount of anesthesia, such as a mild sedative. Once the ultrasound locates the mature follicles in the ovary, the doctor inserts a needle into the follicles and removes the eggs with suction. If the ultrasound can't find or access the ovaries, doctors might have to perform laparoscopic surgery, where doctors make a small incision in the abdomen and locate the ovaries with a tiny fiber-optic lens. This procedure is simple and short, but it requires stronger anesthesia.

3. *Freezing/Vitrification:* Eggs are a little tricky to freeze because of their high water content. Slow freezing could form ice crystals, which could damage the egg when thawed. In a newer process, called vitrification, eggs are placed in a bath with a chemical called cryoprotectant (think of it like anti-freeze), along with sucrose. This helps draw out some of the water and replaces some of it with the cryoprotectant. The eggs are then instantly frozen using liquid nitrogen at −196 degrees.

In 2012, the American Society for Reproductive Medicine announced that egg freezing no longer needed to be labeled as experimental. After reviewing a number of trials comparing fresh and frozen eggs, they concluded that fertility and pregnancy rates were similar with fresh eggs and with eggs frozen by the newer method of vitrification.

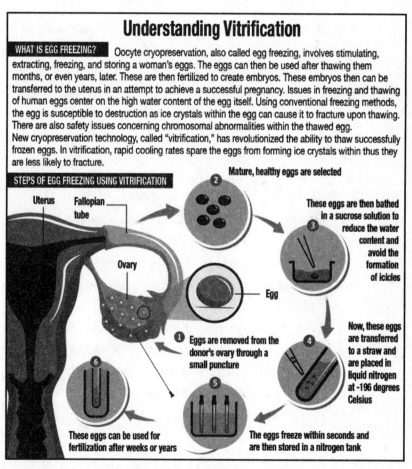

Understanding Vitrification

WHAT IS EGG FREEZING? Oocyte cryopreservation, also called egg freezing, involves stimulating, extracting, freezing, and storing a woman's eggs. The eggs can then be used after thawing them months, or even years, later. These are then fertilized to create embryos. These embryos then can be transferred to the uterus in an attempt to achieve a successful pregnancy. Issues in freezing and thawing of human eggs center on the high water content of the egg itself. Using conventional freezing methods, the egg is susceptible to destruction as ice crystals within the egg can cause it to fracture upon thawing. There are also safety issues concerning chromosomal abnormalities within the thawed egg.

New cryopreservation technology, called "vitrification," has revolutionized the ability to thaw successfully frozen eggs. In vitrification, rapid cooling rates spare the eggs from forming ice crystals within thus they are less likely to fracture.

STEPS OF EGG FREEZING USING VITRIFICATION

Mature, healthy eggs are selected

Uterus   Fallopian tube

Ovary

Egg

These eggs are then bathed in a sucrose solution to reduce the water content and avoid the formation of icicles

① Eggs are removed from the donor's ovary through a small puncture

Now, these eggs are transferred to a straw and are placed in liquid nitrogen at -196 degrees Celsius

⑥ These eggs can be used for fertilization after weeks or years

⑤ The eggs freeze within seconds and are then stored in a nitrogen tank

Source: Mint Research (Used with permission)

Embryo freezing is the most common procedure for preserving fertility. It involves storing embryos before chemotherapy begins. In this procedure, some of your eggs are collected and fertilized by sperm from a spouse, partner, or donor. This process is called *in vitro* fertilization (IVF).

The first steps of embryo freezing are identical to those for egg freezing, ovarian stimulation, and egg retrieval. The next two steps consist of insemination and fertilization and embryo culture.

1. *Insemination:* After retrieval, doctors examine the eggs and decide which of them hold the most potential for a successful pregnancy. They place these eggs in an IVF culture medium to await insemination. Meanwhile, they separate the father's sperm from his semen. The most motile sperm (the "best swimmers") are then added to the eggs in the incubator.

2. *Fertilization and embryo culture:* Usually within a matter of hours, a sperm cell penetrates an egg and fertilizes it. A two- to four-cell embryo appears approximately two days after fertilization. On the third day, a six- to ten-cell embryo is seen. Embryos can be placed in the uterus as early as one day and as late as six days after fertilization. In most cases, they're observed for two to three days to determine if the development is normal.

   The embryos then go through a vitrification process similar to that used to freeze eggs. Your chances of becoming pregnant with a thawed frozen embryo are not affected by the length of time the embryo has been stored.

Unfortunately, some women cannot delay their treatment and do not have the time necessary to undergo ovarian stimulation to create embryos or obtain oocytes for freezing. For these women, ovarian tissue freezing is currently an experimental, outpatient surgical procedure to remove a part of or even a complete ovary. This tissue contains both hormone-producing cells and immature eggs. It is divided into strips and can be frozen for future use through reimplantation or in vitro maturation of eggs.

Ovarian transportation is also known as oophoropexy. In this process the ovaries are repositioned as far as possible from the radiation field before radiation treatments begin. This fertility preservation option has a 79 to 100 percent success rate of protecting ovarian function from the effects of pelvic radiation; however, it does not protect against chemotherapy.

Ovarian suppression is an experimental technique in which a hormone similar to gonadotropin releasing hormone (GnRH) is used to temporarily shut down the ovaries. This places a patient in a menopausal state during chemotherapy. It is done with monthly injections, ideally beginning two to four weeks before chemotherapy. The success rate of ovarian suppression is currently under study. This method does not protect against the effects of radiation. Its most common users are young breast cancer patients at risk of early menopause.

The potentially fertility-sparing technique called radical trachelectomy involves removing the cervix while preserving the uterus for women with early-stage cervical cancer. While fertility is unaffected, several risks remain. Any pregnancy after this procedure is considered high-risk, along with an increased chance of premature birth. This procedure is available only at a limited number of cancer centers.

––––––––––––––––––– MY JOURNEY –––––––––––––––––––

Early menopause is a bitch! Hot flashes, especially during the summer, are just ridiculous, and the roller-coaster ride of emotions can be extremely annoying, especially for anyone else in my orbit. But even worse was the depression, because no one explained beforehand how bad it could be, or how constant. Even long after the cancer is gone, depression and feelings of alienation still follow me—even at the most unexpected times. So the adjustments never cease, and as I grow older, hopefully I'm becoming just a little bit wiser and better able to cope.

Bessie (Birmingham, Alabama)

Late Effects of Hormone Therapy

Hormone therapy with tamoxifen/aromatase inhibitors is usually scheduled for five years. This differs from other treatments, like radiation therapy and chemotherapy, which are completed after a number of weeks or months. Because hormone therapy is taken for a longer period than other treatments, possible side effects and health risks from these medications may also last longer.

Tamoxifen

Tamoxifen is one of a group of drugs called selective estrogen receptor modulators (SERMs), previously mentioned in Chapter 2. It acts like estrogen on some tissues in the body, such as the uterus, but blocks the effects of estrogen on other tissues, such as the breast.

Tamoxifen may cause side effects. Tell your doctor if any of the following symptoms become severe or do not go away:

- Increased bone or tumor pain
- Reddening or pain around the tumor site
- Hot flashes
- Nausea
- Excessive tiredness
- Dizziness
- Depression

- Headache
- Thinning hair
- Weight loss
- Stomach cramps
- Constipation

Rare complications include blood clots in the large veins (deep venous thrombosis), blood clots in the lungs (pulmonary emboli), bone loss (in premenopausal women only), cancer of the uterus (or endometrial cancer), cataracts (clouding of the lens of the eye), and/or stroke.

Dorothy Hamill: BeWisER+ About Breast Cancer

Olympic figure skating gold medal winner Dorothy Hamill was diagnosed with breast cancer in 2008. After undergoing surgery and radiation, she participated in a study conducted at Johns Hopkins University's Kimmel Cancer Center designed to measure the effectiveness of antiestrogen therapies, such as tamoxifen, used to prevent breast cancer from returning.

Although she has remained cancer-free for the past six years, Hamill still suffers side effects from the treatments she received. "Between the hot flashes, achy joints, and fatigue, there was no quality of life," she told *People* magazine.[19] "There were also long-term health risks, such as heart disease and bone loss. I talked to my doctor and determined the best thing would be to get off the medication. Now I want to make sure other women are aware that they may have options."

In 2016, Hamill announced that she has made it her mission to empower other women by helping to launch a national campaign called BeWisER+ About Breast Cancer.[20] The goal of the organization is to help women with estrogen-related breast cancer learn about

---

19. *http://www.people.com/article/dorothy-hamill-breast-cancer-gold-medal*
20. *http://bewiseraboutbreastcancer.org/*

treatment-related side effects and find a personalized treatment plan that's right for them.

Matters of the Heart

Nowadays, more than at any time in our history, people are living longer after a diagnosis of cancer, thanks in part to new therapies and strategies for treatment. But some of the same protocols that help people survive cancer may also damage the heart and lead to cardiovascular problems, including hypertension (high blood pressure), cardiac arrhythmia (heart rhythm problems), and heart failure.

In recent years, the evidence of cardiotoxicities has grown. Investigators from the fields of oncology and cardiology have come together to investigate the biology of these effects and search for ways to prevent, manage, and possibly reverse them. These collaborations have created an entirely new discipline, known as cardio-oncology.

What Is Cardiotoxicity?

The National Cancer Institute defines this term as the "toxicity that affects the heart." This includes not only a direct effect of the drug on the heart but also its effect on peripheral blood vessels due to altered blood flow dynamics or from thrombotic (blood clot) events.

Cardiotoxicity can be manifested in a number of ways:

- *Cardiomyopathy:* The muscles of the heart are weakened and are unable to pump as hard or efficiently as previously.
- *Heart failure:* A condition in which the heart can't pump enough blood to meet the body's needs. In some cases, the heart can't fill with enough blood. In other cases, the heart can't pump blood to the rest of the body with enough force. The most common signs and symptoms of heart failure are shortness

of breath or trouble breathing, fatigue (tiredness), and swelling in the ankles, feet, legs, abdomen, and veins in the neck.

- *Arrhythmias:* Changes in the rhythm of the heartbeat, either faster or slower than usual.
- *Pericarditis:* A condition in which the membrane around the heart is inflamed. This sac is called the pericardium. The most common sign of pericarditis is chest pain. Other symptoms are weakness, palpitations, trouble breathing, and coughing.
- *Thromboembolism:* This refers to blood clots that form in a vein deep in the body, known as deep vein thromboses (DVTs). They occur when blood thickens and clumps together. Although DVTs can occur anywhere in the body, most deep vein blood clots occur in the lower leg or thigh. A blood clot in a deep vein can break off and travel through the bloodstream. The loose clot is called an embolus. It can travel to an artery in the lungs and block blood flow. This condition is called pulmonary embolism, or PE.

Cancer Drugs Can Cause Cardiotoxicity

Anthracyclines drugs (such as daunorubicin, doxorubicin, and epirubicin) are used to treat many types of cancer. They work by damaging the DNA in cancer cells, causing them to die. Anthracyclines can cause heart failure, acute myocarditis (inflammation of the heart muscle itself), or abnormal heart rhythms.

These specific drugs merit further investigation, and we encourage you to check with your doctors as to the overall benefits of their use.

Trastuzumab (Herceptin) is used to treat HER2-positive breast cancer as described in Chapter 2. Like anthracyclines, trastuzumab can cause abnormal heart rhythms and heart failure. Unlike anthracyclines, trastuzumab cardiotoxicity can be reversible.

5-fluorouracil, or 5-FU, is used to treat cancers of the breast, colon, rectum, stomach, and pancreas. It interferes with cancer cells' ability to make DNA. 5-FU can cause angina-like chest pain, heart failure, and cardiogenic shock (when your heart suddenly can't pump enough blood to meet your body's needs), myocardial infarction (heart attack), and even sudden death.

Paclitaxel is used to treat breast and ovarian cancer. It blocks cell growth by stopping cell division and may kill cancer cells. It can cause abnormal heart rhythms, heart failure, and ischemia (inadequate blood supply to an organ or part of the body, including the heart).

Cyclophosphamide (CTX) is used to treat many types of cancer. CTX can cause neuro-hormonal changes, which can push heart dysfunction toward clinical heart failure. It can also cause the mitral valve to leak (mitral regurgitation).

Bevacizumab (Avastin) is used alone or with other drugs to treat certain types of cervical, colorectal, lung, kidney, ovarian, fallopian tube, and primary peritoneal cancer, metastatic breast cancer, and glioblastoma (a type of brain cancer). Bevacizumab prevents the growth of new blood vessels that tumors need to grow and may cause an increase in blood pressure and an increased risk of thrombosis (blood clots).

Checking the Heart Before Treatment

Three factors must be considered in any cancer patient before dealing with the potential cardiotoxic effect of treatment:

1. Detecting patients at the highest risk
2. Developing preventive strategies
3. Early treatment of cardiotoxicity if and when it does appear

Patients with preexisting medical conditions, such as high blood pressure, cardiovascular disease, diabetes, and abnormal cholesterol profiles, may be at higher risk of cardiotoxic effects from chemotherapy/

radiation therapy, and medical management of those conditions may be needed before treatment is started.

It is recommended that all patients undergoing chemotherapy receive a pretreatment heart evaluation, which would assess any preexisting conditions and act as a baseline of heart function. This should start with a personal and family medical history as well as a physical exam, including blood pressure measurement. An electrocardiogram (EKG) can detect any arrhythmias. The most frequently used approach—and most effective—to monitoring heart function is an echocardiogram, a noninvasive technique using sound waves. Research is currently underway to assess whether certain blood tests, which can detect damage to heart muscle cells, will be reliable methods to follow potential cardiotoxicity.

Specific guidelines for follow-up testing have not yet been developed; however, periodic reevaluation of heart function is important to assure the best cardiac outcomes for the ever-increasing number of long-term cancer survivors.

A 2013 study of cardiac problems in women who received radiation therapy for breast cancer found that any exposure of the heart to radiation leads to increases in the risk of ischemic heart disease. Dr. Sarah C. Darby, of the University of Oxford, and her colleagues reported that this effect was greatest for women with a history of heart disease and that women with preexisting cardiac risk factors have "greater absolute increases in risk from radiotherapy than other women."

Chemoprevention of Cardiotoxicity

In May 1995, the U.S. Food and Drug Administration (FDA) approved dexrazoxane hydrochloride for injection (Zinecard) as a treatment to reduce the incidence and severity of cardiomyopathy associated with doxorubicin administration in certain breast cancer patients.

Several clinical trials are exploring new strategies for preventing or reducing damaging cardiovascular changes induced by cancer treatments. An NCI-sponsored study, for instance, will investigate whether carvedilol, a type of drug known as a beta-blocker, can prevent, or possibly reverse, damage to the heart among young adults who received high-dose anthracyclines.

Another clinical trial, sponsored by NHLBI and NCI, is testing whether a statin medication, which is commonly used to treat high cholesterol, can help prevent the cardiotoxic effects of some breast cancer treatments. The Preventing Anthracycline Cardiovascular Toxicity with Statins (PREVENT)[21] trial will investigate whether the use of atorvastatin can help reduce or prevent cardiotoxicity among patients with breast cancer and lymphoma receiving anthracycline treatment.

The identification of other heart protective agents to prevent cardiotoxicity of chemotherapeutic drugs is a high priority for cardio-oncologists.

―――――――――――― **MY JOURNEY** ――――――――――――

When I was first diagnosed with breast cancer, I was scared out of my wits, as I imagine most people are when receiving a cancer diagnosis. I had plenty of sleepless nights, a short fuse, and forgot more than I care to remember. I was worried if they got it all, if it was going to come back, and what other parts of my body were suffering from all the hideous treatment I had to do.

But then something odd began to happen. As I slowly came to determine that I had become a "survivor," I actually began to relax a little. Of course, the doubt is always there, like on any corner I cross I could get run over by a bus. But thirteen years later, I look both ways

―――――――――

21. *https://clinicaltrials.gov/ct2/show/NCT01988571*

before I cross the street and count my blessings. When I get upset about something, I just ask myself, "What if the cancer returned right now? Would this little annoyance be so important?" The answer is always a resounding *no*!

So I sleep pretty good now, and I don't overanalyze every little ache or pain. I mean, by the time you retire, a few things start to hurt, anyway, so I don't sweat any of it. I'm just glad to be here. Simple as pie.

Gabriella (Charlotte, North Carolina)

Two Cancers in One Lifetime?

As the population of cancer survivors continues to grow (over 14.5 million in the United States in 2014 and estimated to rise by 2 percent each year), there is a great need to better understand the long-term health of this population. Nearly one in five cancers diagnosed today occurs in an individual with a previous diagnosis of cancer, and these "second cancers" are a leading cause of morbidity and mortality among cancer survivors. The National Cancer Institute's Surveillance, Epidemiology, and End Results (SEER) program documents that survivors have a 14 percent higher risk of developing a second cancer than would be expected in the general population.

Before proceeding, here are a few definitions to clarify the time line:

- *Primary cancer* is a term used to describe the original (first) tumor in the body. Cancer cells from a primary cancer may spread to other parts of the body and form new or metastatic tumors. These secondary tumors are the same type of cancer as the primary cancer.
- A *second cancer* refers to a completely new primary cancer in a person with a history of cancer.

- *Field cancerization* is a term used to describe the phenomenon in which a cancer patient later gets a second cancer either in the same organ or an organ located near the first cancer. Scientists postulate that the increased risk for this second cancer is that the surrounding tissues were exposed to the same cancer-causing agents as the first cancer. Examples of field cancerization include colorectal, breast, lung, bladder, and head and neck cancers.

Why are cancer survivors at higher risk of a second cancer? The answer is probably a combination of multiple factors, including the following:

- *Lifestyle and environment:* Some cancers are caused by known cancer-producing agents, such as smoking, alcohol, and HPV infection. Smokers can get cancer of the larynx (voice box) but would later also be at risk of getting lung or esophageal cancer. HPV infections can cause cervical infection as well as head and neck cancer.
- *Genetic susceptibility:* As discussed in Chapters 3 and 5, some families pass down abnormal genetic changes, increasing the risk for cancer. The BRAC1 and BRAC2 genes put women (and men) at increased risk for breast cancer and ovarian cancer. Families with Lynch syndrome (discussed in Chapter 7) have an increased risk for cancers of the stomach, small intestine, liver, gallbladder ducts, upper urinary tract, brain, and skin.

Previous cancer treatments may also increase a patient's risk of a second cancer. They include:

Radiation Therapy

Exposure to radiation has been known for many years as a potential cause of cancer, going back to the study of survivors of the atomic bomb blasts in Japan. Workers exposed to radiation in their jobs and cancer patients who have received radiotherapy are also at higher risk of cancer caused by their exposure.

Many kinds of blood as well as solid tumors can be linked to previous radiation therapy. Several kinds of leukemia, including acute myelogenous leukemia (AML), chronic myelogenous leukemia (CML), and acute lymphoblastic leukemia (ALL), as well as a bone marrow cancer called myelodysplastic syndrome (see the story of Robin Roberts) can all be caused by previous radiation exposure. The increase in risk is dependent on the amount of radiation the bone marrow received during treatment. These cancers tend to occur within a few years after radiation therapy, typically within five to nine years after exposure.

Solid tumors, which are caused by radiation therapy, tend to occur much later, perhaps even ten to fifteen years or more after exposure. The risk is dependent on the dose of radiation, the patient's age at the time of treatment (higher risk in younger patients), and the area where the radiation was given. Some organs, such as breast and thyroid, are more sensitive to the effects than others.

Chemotherapy

This has also been linked to second cancers. The most common cancers linked to chemotherapy are myelodysplastic syndrome (MDS) and AML. Some patients develop MDS, which later turns into AML. The risk of these cancers is higher with chemotherapy than with radiation therapy.

Alkylating agents, such as mechlorethamine, chlorambucil, cyclophosphamide (Cytoxan), melphalan, lomustine (CCNU), carmustine (BCNU), and busulfan are all known to cause leukemia and MDS. Higher drug dose and dose intensity as well as longer therapy duration increase the risk of leukemia. The risk is greatest beginning two years after treatment and reaches its peak five to ten years after exposure.

Other chemotherapeutic drugs known to cause leukemia include cisplatin and carboplatin, as well as a class of drugs called topoisomerase II inhibitors. They work by stopping cancer cells from being able to repair DNA. One subset of topoisomerase II inhibitors called anthracyclines is less likely to cause leukemia. However, as previously mentioned, they can have toxic effects on the heart.

Stem Cell Transplant

This is a method of giving chemotherapy and replacing blood-forming cells destroyed by the treatment. Stem cells (immature blood cells) are removed from the blood or bone marrow of a donor and frozen for storage. Patients then receive high doses of chemotherapy/radiation therapy. Upon completion, the stored stem cells are thawed and replaced in the patient through an infusion. These reinfused stem cells grow into (and restore) the body's blood cells.

Any type of stem cell transplant puts a patient at increased risk of second cancer because of the chemo and radiation therapy received. In addition, patients who receive stem cells from a donor will need to be on drugs to suppress their immune system to prevent rejection of the donor's stem cells. As some cells of the immune system recognize cancer cells as abnormal and kill them, immune suppressive drugs can decrease this ability.

Robin Roberts: Making News

Good Morning America anchor Robin Roberts was diagnosed with breast cancer in 2007. She underwent surgery, chemotherapy, and six weeks of radiation therapy. Despite this, she returned to the anchor desk only a couple of weeks after having her surgery, wearing a wig because she "didn't want to distract viewers from the news."

In 2012, Roberts became concerned about an extreme level of

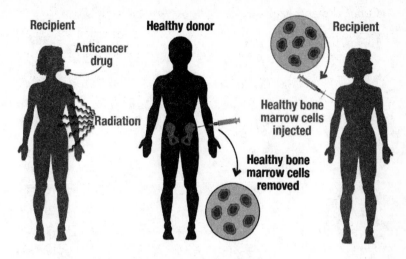

Recipient   Healthy donor   Recipient

Anticancer drug

Radiation

Healthy bone marrow cells injected

Healthy bone marrow cells removed

Allogeneic Stem Cell Transplant

fatigue she was experiencing, more than she had ever previously felt because of her early morning wake-up. She had blood tests and a bone marrow biopsy and was diagnosed with a disorder called myelo-dysplastic syndrome (MDS). These are a group of diseases in which the bone marrow does not make enough healthy blood cells, and researchers think that it may have been the result of the radiation or chemotherapy Roberts received to treat her breast cancer.

It was determined in 2012 that she needed a stem cell transplant. Robin's sister, Sally Ann Roberts, an anchor for WWL-TV in New Orleans, was an excellent match and became the bone marrow donor. Before the actual procedure, Robin Roberts had to undergo ten days of intense chemotherapy to remove any abnormal cells from her body before the new immune cells were introduced. Five months to the day after her bone marrow transplant in 2012, Robin Roberts triumphantly returned to her place at the anchor desk on *Good Morning America*.

The Case of Robin Roberts and the Need for Minority Donors

In June 2012, in a show of support for their colleague Robin Roberts, *Good Morning America* promoted bone marrow donation by sponsoring a bone marrow registry drive at ABC studios in New York. *GMA*'s George Stephanopoulos and Lara Spencer, as well as ABC News president Ben Sherwood showed up at the drive and had their cheeks swabbed to join the registry.

According to Jeffrey Chell, CEO of Be The Match,[22] over 44,000 people have registered with the National Marrow Donor Program (NMDR) since Roberts announced her diagnosis. This is over 20,000 more than the registry would normally receive in that period! It is estimated that sixty to seventy of these new donors will be a good match and have their marrow used in a transplant.

However, Robin Roberts's bone marrow transplant also highlights a more pressing problem, which is an acute shortage of minority donors. Because of this, the chance of finding a match on the national registry is as low as 76 percent for African Americans and other minorities, compared with 97 percent for Caucasians.

Of the over 9 million potential donors in the Be The Match registry, Caucasians constitute nearly three-quarters of the donors. Hispanics are at 10 percent and Asians and African Americans are at 7 percent each. As HLA typing tends to be closest within racial groups, this can make finding a suitable donor a difficult proposition.

In multiracial populations, the problem is even more acute. According to the 2010 census, the multiracial population among American children has increased almost 50 percent since 2000. This makes it the fastest growing youth group in the country.

Programs have been established to increase awareness in communities with a special emphasis on African Americans, American Indian/

---

22. *https://bethematch.org/*

Alaskan Natives, Asian/Pacific Islanders, and Hispanics. One of these is the National MOTTEP[23] (National Minority Organ and Tissue Transplant Education Program), whose mission is to educate ethnic minority Americans about the need for organ, tissue, and blood donations. MOTTEP simultaneously educates communities about the diseases and behaviors that lead to the need for transplantation.

What's a Single Mother to Do?

According to a 2010 study published in the journal *Cancer*, more than 1.5 million parents in the United States who are being treated for some form of cancer are also raising minor children, and approximately 25 percent of them are single parents. This challenge is even more prevalent among African American women, who, according to the U.S. Census Bureau, are most likely to be single parents (68 percent of black women who gave birth in 2011 were unmarried, compared with 36 percent overall) and are most inclined to be diagnosed with breast cancer at a young age, when it can be more aggressive.

Alexia Elejalde-Ruiz reported in the *Chicago Tribune* on September 25, 2013, that a 1996 study published in the journal *Cancer Practice* found that single mothers with breast cancer had significantly higher rates of depression than married women, and reported higher numbers of illness-related pressures on their families. Their children scored in the abnormal range on measures of self-worth and acceptance.

University of Washington School of Nursing professor Frances Marcus Lewis, the lead author on that study, found that single mothers "struggle with a huge sense of personal vulnerability, which is beyond what we have seen among women who are married or unhappily married."

---

23. *http://www.nationalmottep.org/*

Cancer survivor and founder and executive director of Along Comes Hope, Jenny Mulks Wieneke, agrees. "It is a natural instinct to protect your child at all costs," she says, "even when you've been diagnosed with cancer and a potential death sentence. How do you protect your child when your own world is being shattered? When I was diagnosed, the doctor put her thumb and forefinger together and showed me an inch, which was her answer to my question about my chances of survival."

Jenny, like many other mothers, found her family life thrown immediately into crisis mode when she received her cancer diagnosis. She was forced into a role she had no idea how to fill. As a single mother, many women represent an all-encompassing security blanket for their children, and a diagnosis of cancer will surely cause that world to spin off its axis. "The most important thing I could do was share with Gabriel, on his four-year-old level, what we were facing. The challenge was finding a balance between sharing every detail and only what he needed to know to prepare for what we were facing."

The best way to determine this is by first considering the age and maturity of your children. What can they understand and how is their personality suited to handle adversity? "I was told that I had little hope of surviving past a year," Jenny says. "Sharing that with him was beyond his scope of comprehension, and mine, too, for that matter. Children have an innate gift of hope and live in a land of 'what ifs.' When it comes to capturing that magical spirit of hope and not letting another person predetermine your fate, we can learn a lot from them."

So what's a mother to do? Most children are used to seeing their parents in a position of strength, capable of taking care of things on a daily basis. But then cancer shows up, and they may see their favorite adult person become vulnerable, scared, and sick. This is such a crucial time to continue the dialogue that will become part of the healing journey for all parties—to heal, to fight, and to find love and hope along the way.

"My vulnerability brought about different behaviors in Gabriel," Jenny says. "He became my brave little helper. He also became quite fearful of losing me, asking if I was going to die, which created a long-term fear of abandonment. Because of the fragility of his emotional state, my treatment strategy became very difficult. I had no chance to survive where we were in California, but going to MD Anderson in Houston, Texas, meant a yearlong commitment—if I survived. And when you've been told you have maybe a year to live, the *last* thing you want to do is roll the dice for a chance to survive when it means leaving your child! I only wanted to be with him. So while it broke my heart to leave home, he was the light I was reaching for by taking this chance to survive."

Jenny, like many other women, had an impossible choice to make, especially when facing death as a very real possibility. "Coming home to Gabriel was what kept me going through such tough treatment," Jenny says. "Death was simply not an option. Choosing a treatment plan is difficult, but in my case, since I was putting everything on the line, I opted for the most aggressive plan I could."

But Jenny faced what many other parents must contend with if they have young children. Until they reach a certain age, children have little concept of time, and a week may seem like an impossibly long time, prompting great fears that a parent may never return. "Because of this, I created the Mommy Box," Jenny explains. "If I had to be gone for seven nights, I left seven little toys individually wrapped inside the box. Each morning before preschool, I got on the phone with Gabriel and he would go pick out a gift from the box, excitedly unwrap it, and tell me what it was. Day by day, the gifts would dwindle, and on the last morning, when there were no more gifts in the box, he knew that it meant I was coming home and I would be his gift. Needless to say, as my treatment progressed, I had many backup gifts I'd wrap up just in case I became delayed getting home. This really helped him understand time and to trust that I would return."

While every mother may not be able to engineer a Mommy Box for her child, she will inevitably find ways to provide comfort and trust and hope. Fortunately, Jenny's cancer was treatable, and her son managed without her, with the great help of family and friends.

Gabriel is now thirteen years old. He and Jenny still talk about his Mommy Box and some of the treasures he received. "I think the biggest takeaway from it was the sense of security and love it made him feel in knowing I was ultimately coming home each time the Mommy Box appeared. A four-year-old is going to ask you point-blank if you're going to die, and you need to answer that. You need to acknowledge their fear and share your fear, as well. On the other hand, a thirteen-year-old will think about you dying and probably not ask you if you're going to die, but you need to be proactive in bringing it up and sharing where you are in this journey."

As we've learned from Jenny and many others, cancer affects the entire family, which means communicating is the key to surviving—to living and learning and loving your way through it—together.

Survivorship and Quality of Life

Of the more than 15 million cancer survivors on record in the United States in 2014, nearly a quarter of them were originally diagnosed with breast cancer. Considering the increase in the number of long-term survivors due to advances in early detection and treatment, it is imperative that we enhance our understanding of the dynamics of long-term survivorship and how it affects the whole person, not just their physical symptoms and health but their overall quality of life.

The *European Journal of Cancer* urged in 2005 that because of the growing numbers of long-term breast cancer survivors, specific treatments needed to be adapted in order to accommodate and support this trend. Their research showed that women who survived longer after a diagnosis of breast cancer reported a better overall quality of life and better psychological and social well-being than women with fewer years of survival.

Since then, studies of breast cancer patients have continued to find that when psychosocial care is added to a patient's general treatment, her short- *and* long-term quality of life may be significantly improved, especially compared with women who did not receive this intervention.

On another front, it has also been proven that psychosocial care not only improves a woman's health. Studies show that it also reduces healthcare billings by 24 percent in women who attended psychosocial intervention projects compared with women who did not.[24]

According to a 1997 review article in *Oncology* by Betty R. Ferrell, PhD, RN, and Karen Hassey Dow, PhD, RN, "Quality of life (QOL) issues have become a vital area of concern to cancer survivors, their families, and care providers" and "future advances in cancer treatment will further heighten the importance of survivorship issues in comprehensive cancer care."

These issues began to come to the forefront beginning in 1990 when the National Cancer Institute (NCI) began using QOL measures to compare treatments, as well as having them serve as markers for treatment trials, general assessors of rehabilitation needs, and predictors of future responses to a variety of treatments. The NCI continues to expand its use of QOL controls in clinical trials, research, and outcome studies, with a special emphasis to assess QOL in culturally diverse populations.

---

24. *https://www.researchgate.net/publication/7540830*

An increasing number of cancer centers throughout the country are increasing their resources to support and treat the long-term implications of cancer treatment, in particular the consequences faced by women dealing with gender-specific cancers.

In the next chapter, we will explore a wide range of conventional and complementary treatments that address many of these issues.

KEY POINTS TO REMEMBER

✓ More than 150,000 American women are diagnosed each year with cancer during their reproductive years (younger than age forty-five).

✓ One in four people with cancer reports memory and attention problems after chemotherapy.

✓ Dealing with cancer can lead to serious depression, severe emotional distress, and interference with sleep.

✓ Modern technology has allowed many women to preserve their fertility.

✓ Early menopause can occur in any woman undergoing cancer treatment, even in those who have not had their ovaries removed.

✓ Patients with preexisting medical conditions may be at higher risk of cardiotoxic effects from chemotherapy/ radiation therapy.

✓ All patients receiving chemotherapy should have a pretreatment heart evaluation.

THE WORST POEM EVER

I suck doing poems of dying and pain,
I suck when I'm trying to write in the rain.

I suck when you cut me.
I suck when I heal.

I suck doing chemo.
I suck deep for real.

I just suck.

I want so bad to write the perfect words,
with just the right bounce of heart and pace.

I want to say all those things one says,
when the day goes dark and the lights go out.

Oh! That's when things go deep with meaning.

I can lay here in peace on my bed of nails,
still and content just to be here, alive.

I got no rhymes, no more to give,
no love songs or neat turns of phrase.

I just got this worst poem ever
and a big bad burning will to live.

—Anonymous

12

CONVENTIONAL AND COMPLEMENTARY WISDOM: Managing the Side Effects of Cancer Treatment

Thoughts and consciousness are pivotal
in creating a healing environment in the body.
With hope we can get closer to that day
when that wolf named cancer is quiet,
still and powerless.

—Gwyneth Paltrow from *Stand Up to Cancer*

What's New?

In Chapters 10 and 11, we discussed many of the residual issues affecting women during a cancer journey. Now we'd like to help you manage as many of those short- and long-term side effects as possible.

When someone is diagnosed with cancer, she wants to do everything possible to combat the disease as well as manage its symptoms and cope with any consequences of treatment. Many turn to complementary health options, including natural products, such as herbs and dietary supplements; medical marijuana; and mind-body practices, including acupuncture, massage, and yoga; as well as writing and an assortment of art therapy.

This introductory overview of these approaches is based on collaboration between the U.S. National Center for Complementary and Integrative Health (NCCIH) and the U.S. National Cancer Institute (NCI). These options have been studied either for cancer prevention, treatment of the disease, or symptom management. We'll include what the science says about their effectiveness as well as any concerns about their safety.

Anemia

This condition refers to a lower than normal red blood cell count, which most often leads to fatigue, along with pale skin in some people.

Here's what we recommend:

Save your energy. Don't be afraid to ask for help. Figure out your most important tasks for the day, and when people offer to help, let them do so. They can take you to the doctor, empty the dishwasher, make meals, or do other things you are too tired to do.

Balance rest with activity. Take short naps during the day, but keep in mind that too much bed rest can make you feel weak. You may feel better if you take short walks or exercise a little every day. Even five minutes of activity here and there can do wonders.

Eat and drink well. You may need to eat foods that are high in protein or iron. Your doctor, nurse, or a registered dietitian can help decide what foods are best for you. The familiar adage "you are what you eat" could not be more accurate when it comes to treating and preventing disease—of *any* kind.

> **NOTE to PATIENT:**
> If you have cancer, seek nutritional counseling.

Loss of Appetite

Take these steps to ensure that you are getting the nutrition you need to stay strong during and after treatment:

Drink plenty of liquids. Losing fluid can lead to dehydration, a dangerous condition. You may become weak or dizzy and have dark yellow urine if you are not drinking enough liquids.

Choose healthy and high-nutrient foods. Eat a little, even if you are not hungry. Have five or six small meals throughout the day instead of three large meals. Try to eat nutrient-dense foods that are high in protein and calories. Keep a supply of tasty quality protein bars on hand.

Stay active. Movement will actually increase your appetite. Even taking a short walk each day can help. Taking one of those protein bars with you when you're out—along with a bottle of water—will come in handy.

Bleeding and Bruising

Take these steps if you are at increased risk of bleeding and bruising:

Avoid certain medicines. Many over-the-counter medicines contain aspirin or ibuprofen, which can increase your risk of bleeding. When in doubt, check the label. You may also be advised to limit or avoid alcohol if your platelet count is low.

Take extra care to prevent bleeding. Brush your teeth gently, with a very soft toothbrush. Wear shoes, even when you are inside. Be extra careful when using sharp objects. Use an electric shaver instead of a razor. Use lotion and a lip balm to prevent dry, chapped skin and lips.

Tell your doctor or nurse if you are constipated or notice bleeding from your rectum. If you do start to bleed, press down firmly on the area with a clean cloth. Keep pressing until the bleeding stops. If you bruise, put ice on the area.

―――――――――― MY JOURNEY ――――――――――

Cancer has caused me to depend on other people in ways I never previously imagined. I was always a self-sufficient person and didn't even know how to ask for help. So when I became perpetually tired during treatment, I had to suck it up and basically beg. Once I did, I couldn't stop. And the remarkable thing is, I think my friends actually *liked* helping me!

Shanaya (St. Louis, Missouri)

Constipation

Follow these tips to prevent or treat constipation:

Eat high-fiber foods. Adding bran to food, such as cereals or smoothies, is an easy way to get more fiber in your diet.

Drink plenty of liquids. Most people need to drink at least eight cups of liquid each day. You may require more based upon the climate you live in, as well as your treatment, medications you are taking, or other health factors. Drinking warm or hot liquids may also help.

Try to be active every day. Most people can do light exercise, even in a bed or chair. Other people choose to walk, or ride an exercise bike, for fifteen to thirty minutes each day.

Use medicines and treatments prescribed by your doctor. Some over-the-counter products may lead to bleeding, infection, or other harmful side effects.

Diarrhea

Following are ideas to prevent complications from diarrhea:

Drink plenty of fluid each day. Diarrhea causes the body to lose fluids rapidly, and dehydration could develop if you're not drinking enough water.

Eat small meals. This is easier on your stomach and digestive system. For most people, foods high in potassium and sodium (minerals lost when you have diarrhea) are good choices.

Check with your doctor or nurse before taking medicine. Your doctor will prescribe the correct diarrhea medicine for you.

Keep your anal area clean and dry. Use warm water and wipes to stay clean. It may help to take warm, shallow baths (sitz baths).

Fatigue

This is a common side effect of many cancer treatments, including chemotherapy, radiation therapy, biological therapy, bone marrow transplant, and surgery. Co-conditions such as anemia, as well as pain, medications, and emotions can also cause or worsen fatigue.

People often describe cancer-related fatigue as feeling extremely tired, weak, heavy, run-down, and having no energy. Resting does not always help with cancer-related fatigue. This is one of the most difficult side effects to cope with for many people.

Try some of these solutions:

Make a plan that balances rest and activity. Choose relaxing activities. For example, listen to music, write, read, meditate, practice guided imagery, or spend time with people you enjoy. Any of these can preserve energy and lower stress. Your doctor may also advise light exercise to give you more energy and help you feel better. If you do get tired, take short naps (less than an hour) during the day. Too much sleep during the day can make it difficult to sleep enough at night.

Eat and drink well. Foods high in protein and calories will help you maintain your strength. Eat several small meals throughout the day instead of three big meals. Stay well hydrated. Limit your intake of caffeine and alcohol.

Meet with a specialist. It may help to meet with a counselor, psychologist, or psychiatrist. These experts help people to cope with difficult thoughts and feelings. Lowering stress may give you more energy. Since uncontrolled pain can also be major source of fatigue, it may help to meet with a pain or palliative care specialist.

> **NOTE to PATIENT:**
> Palliative care is not specifically end-of-life care.
> It offers you a plan to manage pain and
> can be quite temporary.

Hair Loss

For those receiving chemo or radiation therapy, hair can fall out slowly or seemingly overnight, depending on a number of factors. But no matter how it happens, there are ways to manage it.

Treat your hair gently. You may choose a hairbrush with soft bristles or a wide-tooth comb. Do not use hair dryers, irons, or products such as gels or clips that may hurt your scalp. Wash your hair less often and with a mild shampoo. Be very gentle. Pat it dry with a soft towel.

Shorten or shave? Some people choose to cut their hair short to make it easier to deal with when it starts to fall out. Others choose to shave their heads. If you choose to shave your head, use an electric shaver so you won't cut yourself. If you plan to buy a wig, get one while you still have hair so you can match it to your current or natural color. If you find wigs to be itchy and hot, try wearing a comfortable scarf or turban.

Protect and care for your scalp. Use sunscreen or wear a hat when you are outside. Choose something comfortable that you enjoy and keeps your head warm. If your scalp itches or feels tender, lotions and conditioners (without harsh chemicals) can help it feel better.

Anger, depression, and embarrassment are all common reactions to hair loss. It can help to share these feelings with someone who understands. Some people find it helpful to write down their feelings and/or talk with other people who have lost their hair during cancer treatment.

Will It Grow Back?

Yes. After chemotherapy treatment has ended, hair often grows back in two to three months. It will be very fine when it starts growing again. Sometimes, it can be curlier or straighter—or even a different color or shade—than it was prior to loss. Eventually, it may return to how it was before treatment.

After radiation therapy has ended, hair usually grows back within three to six months. If you received a very high dose of radiation, your hair may grow back thinner or not at all on the part of your body that received radiation.

In any case, no matter what type of treatment you received, be gentle with your hair when it begins growing back. Avoid too much brushing, curling, and blow-drying. You may not want to wash your hair as frequently, either, until it begins to feel stronger. Avoid shampoos and conditioners with harsh chemicals, and definitely stay away from coloring your hair unless you are 100 percent sure the dye is chemical-free and safe for use.

From now on, mild, organic products are your best option.

―――――――――――――― MY JOURNEY ――――――――――――――

I started chemo in September, right around the time Halloween costumes were going on sale everywhere. My hair fell out within the first month, and I wasn't prepared with even a headscarf, let alone a wig. I didn't own a hat except for a stupid pillbox thing I once wore to a friend's wedding. The closest place that sold any decent wigs was miles away. What was I going to do? Buy a Halloween costume with a cheap wig, or try to find one online? I decided to stay bald and see what happened.

It sure became a conversation starter, but not one I always welcomed. I mean, how many times can people stare at you and say how sorry they are? Boring. One day, when I was especially fed up with people trying to be so sensitive and caring about my losing my hair, I blurted, "No, I haven't lost my hair. I just made it go away in your mind!" This woman just stood there open-mouthed until I told her I was kidding, that it really was gone, and that I could make hers go away, too, if she wanted, because it saves so much money on shampoo and conditioner and haircuts and all the rest of the ridiculous things we do for our hair. Well, she laughed, and I did, too, and then I went home and bought a wig online.

Clarissa (Palmer, Massachusetts)

Preventing Infection

When it comes to hygiene, common sense is a good place to begin, but there are a few more factors to keep in mind during treatment:

Wash your hands often and well. Use soap and warm water, especially before eating. Have people around you wash their hands, too.

Stay extra clean. If you have a catheter, keep the area around it clean and dry. Brush your teeth well and check your mouth each day for sores or other signs of infection. If you get a scrape or cut, clean it well. Let your doctor or nurse know if your bottom is sore or bleeds, as this can increase your risk of infection.

Avoid human germs. Stay away from people who are sick or have a cold. Avoid crowds and people who have just had a live vaccine, such as one for chicken pox, polio, or measles. As people in some parts of Asia often do when they are sick and out and about, consider wearing a breathable face mask if you're travelling in a crowded environment, like a subway or train.

Monitor your food hygiene. Follow food safety guidelines by making sure that the meat, fish, and eggs you eat are well-cooked. Keep hot foods hot and cold foods cold. You may be advised to eat only fruits and vegetables that can be peeled, or to wash all raw fruits and vegetables very well. In fact, it's always wise to thoroughly wash any type of raw food.

─────────────── **MY JOURNEY** ───────────────

It was terribly hot when I first underwent radiation therapy. I had a very abstract painting that reminded me of Salvador Dali drawn on my chest to remind everyone where I was supposed to get cooked, and they told me to keep the area dry for the next two months. That was definitely a challenge—one that I felt like I was failing almost every time I took a shower. I wasn't supposed to wear deodorant either, at least not the kind one usually finds in the average pharmacy, because the artificial ingredients would irritate me. Finally, after asking around, I discovered a product made from seaweed and a bunch of other organic minerals. My doctor balked at first but eventually relented. In this case, I taught *him* something he didn't already know, and I made it through the summer a lot more comfortable.

Kris (Jacksonville, Florida)

Lymphedema

These steps may help prevent lymphedema or keep it from getting worse:

Protect your skin. Use lotion to avoid dry skin, and use sunscreen. Consider wearing plastic gloves with cotton lining when working in order to prevent scratches, cuts, or burns. Keep your feet clean and dry. Keep your nails clean and short to prevent ingrown nails and infection. Avoid tight shoes and wear your jewelry loose.

Exercise. Work to keep body fluids moving, especially in places where lymphedema has developed. Start with gentle exercises that help you move and contract your muscles. Ask your doctor or nurse or physical therapist about which exercises are best for you.

Manual lymph drainage. See a trained specialist (a certified lymphedema therapist) to receive a type of therapeutic massage called manual lymph drainage. Therapeutic massage works best to lower lymphedema when given early, before symptoms progress.

Memory and Concentration Problems

It's important for you or a family member to tell your health-care team if you have difficulty remembering things, thinking, or concentrating. Take these steps to help manage minor memory or concentration problems:

Plan your day. Do things that require the most concentration during the time of day when you feel best. Get extra rest and plenty of sleep at night. If you need rest during the day, short naps of less than one hour are best. Maintain a daily routine as best as you can.

Exercise your body and mind. Exercise can help to decrease stress and keep you feeling more alert. Exercise releases endorphins, also known as "feel-good chemicals," which provide feelings of positivity. Mind-body practices, like meditation, or mental exercises, such as puzzles or games, can also help some people.

Write down—and keep handy—a list of important information. Use a daily planner, recorder, or other electronic device to help you remember important activities. Make a list of important names and phone numbers. Keep it in one place so it's easy to find.

And while you're at it, take time to expand your writing into areas of self-expression, as it's important to get in touch with your feelings during this stressful time.

Mouth and Throat Problems

Cancer treatments are notorious for creating problems in the mouth and throat. Here are a few ideas to help ease those challenges.

For a sore mouth or throat, choose foods that are soft, wet, and easy to swallow. Soften dry foods with gravy, sauce, or other liquids. Use a blender to make milkshakes or blend your food to make it easier to swallow. Ask about pain medicine, such as lozenges or sprays, that numb your mouth and make eating less painful. Avoid food and drinks that can irritate your mouth, i.e., foods that are crunchy, salty, spicy, or sugary, as well as alcoholic drinks. And, it should go without saying, do not smoke or use tobacco products.

For a dry mouth, drink plenty of liquids because a dry mouth can increase the risk of tooth decay and mouth infections. Keep water handy and sip it often to keep your mouth wet. Suck on ice chips or sugar-free hard candy, eat frozen desserts, or chew sugar-free gum. Use a lip balm. Ask about medicines such as saliva substitutes that can coat, protect, and moisten your mouth and throat. Acupuncture may also help with dry mouth.

Changes to your sense of taste may make foods seem tasteless or not taste the way they used to. Radiation therapy may cause a change in sweet, sour, bitter, and salty tastes. Chemotherapy drugs may cause an unpleasant chemical or metallic taste in your mouth. If you experience taste changes, try different foods to find ones that taste best to you. Eating cold foods may also help.

Here are some more tips to consider to help you with changing tastes:

- If food tastes bland, marinate before cooking to improve flavor, or add mild spices.
- If red meat—even in suggested limited amounts—tastes strange, switch to other high-protein foods, such as chicken, eggs, fish, peanut butter, turkey, beans, or certain dairy products.
- If foods taste salty, bitter, or acidic, try sweetening them with a bit of honey.
- If foods taste metallic, switch to plastic utensils and nonmetal cooking dishes.
- If you have a bad taste in your mouth, try sugar-free lemon drops, gum, or mints.

> **NOTE to PATIENT:**
> Consult with a cancer-friendly nutritionist!

———— MY JOURNEY ————

It started with a little mouth sore. I used a load of Listerine and they eventually went away. Then my nose started growing things—inside, where nobody could see, but I could *feel*, and it was no picnic. I live in a dry climate, but still, this was too much! My nose was bleeding every day. One nurse suggested a humidifier, which helped a little. That's just the neck up. Don't get me started on everything below.

Liz (Manchester, New Hampshire)

Nausea and Vomiting

What may have been a badge of honor during high school or college is nothing to laugh about when it comes to feeling sick during cancer treatment. Here are some suggestions to ease these troublesome side effects.

Take antinausea medicine, which your doctor can prescribe. Most people need to take an antinausea medicine even on days when they feel well. Tell your doctor or nurse if the medicine you're taking doesn't help. Different options may work better for you.

Drink plenty of water and fluids to prevent dehydration. Make a habit of sipping water/tea throughout the day. Be careful to avoid drinks with high sugar content.

Avoid foods that are greasy, fried, sweet, or spicy. This will help, especially if you feel sick after eating them. If the smell of food bothers you while cooking, ask others to make your food. Try cold foods that do not have strong smells, or let food cool down before you eat it.

Eat a small snack before treatment. This can help many people handle those days a little easier. Others avoid eating or drinking right before or after treatment because it makes them feel sick. After treatment, wait at least one hour before you eat or drink.

Learn about complementary medicine practices. For some, acupuncture relieves nausea/vomiting caused by chemotherapy. Deep breathing, guided imagery, hypnosis, and other relaxation techniques (such as listening to music, reading a book, or meditating) may also help. Read more about these options later in this chapter.

Nerves and Senses

If you have experienced nerve changes, you may be advised to take these steps:

Prevent falls. Move rugs so you will not trip on them. Ask for help with this, if needed. Put rails on walls and especially in the bathroom so you can hold on to them for balance and security. Put bath mats in the shower or tub. Wear sturdy shoes with soft soles. Get up slowly after sitting or lying down, especially if you feel dizzy.

Take extra care in the kitchen and shower. Use potholders in the kitchen to protect your hands from burns. Be careful when handling knives or sharp objects. Ask someone to check the water temperature to make sure it's not too hot.

Protect your hands and feet. Wear shoes indoors and out. Check your arms, legs, and feet daily for cuts or scratches. If it's cold, wear warm clothes to protect your hands and feet.

Ask for help and slow down. Let people help you with difficult tasks. Slow down and give yourself more time to do things.

Ask about pain medicine and integrative medicine practices. You may be prescribed pain medicine. Other methods, such as acupuncture, massage, physical therapy, and yoga, may also lessen pain. Talk with your healthcare team to learn what is best for you. You can find more about these later in this chapter.

The Pain Game

Here is a guide for you and your healthcare team to prevent, treat, or lessen pain.

Keep track of your pain profile. Each day write about any pain you feel. Specify where it hurts and describe the pain (sharp, burning, shooting, or throbbing). What triggers the pain, and how long does it last? Does it interfere with desired activities, such as eating, sleeping, or working? What makes it feel better—or worse? For example, do ice packs, heating pads, or exercises help? Does pain medicine help, and how much do you take and how often? Rate your pain on a scale of one to ten, with one signifying the least and ten the most.

Take pain medicine as prescribed. Don't wait until your pain becomes severe before taking your meds. That can delay relief. Tell your doctor or nurse if the medicine is no longer effective, or if the pain returns before it is time to take the next dose.

Consider meeting with a pain specialist, who often works together with a pain or palliative care team and may include a neurologist, surgeon, physiatrist, psychiatrist, psychologist, or pharmacist.

Ask about integrative medicine. Treatments such as acupuncture, biofeedback, hypnosis, massage therapy, and physical therapy may help treat pain and are discussed later in this chapter.

─────────────── **MY JOURNEY** ───────────────

Nobody told me about how my thighs would get fried from radiation or how they would hurt so bad I could hardly walk or sit down. I was able to ease the pain at home with a lot of ointment, but what was I supposed to do at work or anywhere else? I called my oncologist, begging for pain meds, which got me through the worst of it. But I couldn't call every time I was hurting or else I would have never gotten off the phone and would have driven her office crazy. I found out that the worst side effects eventually recede.

Patti (Buffalo, New York)

Skin Care

Depending on what treatment you are receiving, a host of options are available to protect your skin, prevent infection, and reduce itching.

Use mild soaps that are gentle on your skin. Ask for specific recommendations for lotions and creams, and ask if you should avoid any skin products. For example, you may be advised not to use powders or antiperspirants before radiation therapy.

Protect your skin. Lotions or antibiotics may be needed for dry, itchy, infected, or swollen skin. Avoid heating pads, ice packs, or bandages on areas receiving radiation therapy. Shave less often and use an electric razor—or stop shaving—if your skin is sore. When outdoors, wear sunscreen and lip balm, loose fitting pants and long-sleeved shirts, and a wide-brimmed hat.

Prevent or treat dry, itchy skin (pruritus). Avoid products with alcohol or perfume, which can dry or irritate your skin. Take short showers or baths in lukewarm water. Put on lotion after pat drying off from a shower, while your skin is still slightly damp. Keep your home cool and humid. Eat a healthy diet and drink plenty of fluids to keep your skin moist and healthy. Applying a cool washcloth or ice to the affected area may also help. Consider acupuncture, too.

Prevent or treat minor nail problems. Keep your nails clean and cut short. Wear gloves when you wash dishes, work in the garden, or clean the house.

Sleep Issues

If you're having trouble falling—or staying— asleep, consider these helpful steps:

Tell your doctor about problems that interfere with sleep. Getting treatment to deal with those issues (such as pain or bladder or gastro-intestinal problems) may help you sleep better.

Cognitive behavioral therapy (CBT) and relaxation therapy may help. A CBT therapist can help you learn to change negative thoughts and beliefs about sleep into positive ones. Strategies such as muscle relaxation, guided imagery, and self-hypnosis may also help.

Set good bedtime habits. Go to bed only when sleepy in a quiet, dark room in a comfortable bed. If you do not fall asleep, get out of bed then return to bed when you are sleepy. Stop watching television or using other electrical devices a couple of hours before going to bed. Don't drink or eat a lot before bedtime. While it's important to keep active during the day with regular exercise, exercising within a few hours before bedtime may make sleep more difficult.

If other strategies do not work, your doctor may prescribe sleep medicine for a short period. The sleep medicine prescribed will depend on your specific problem (such as trouble falling asleep or trouble staying asleep) as well as other medicines you are taking.

Urinary Symptoms

It's never a bad idea to remind ourselves about staying hydrated, so let's begin with that and add a few other thoughts that contribute to good urinary health.

Drink enough liquid. Urine should be light yellow or clear. Avoid things that can make bladder problems worse, like caffeine, drinks with alcohol, spicy foods, and tobacco products.

Lower your chances of getting a urinary tract infection. Go often to the bathroom. Wear cotton underwear and loose-fitting pants. Learn about safe and sanitary practices for catheterization, and take showers instead of baths.

——————————— MY JOURNEY ———————————

Whenever something bad happens, like I lose my umbrella, the stock market dives a little, or my car dies, I just say to myself, "Baby, it could be *way* worse! You could still have cancer!" So I'm good.

Not too much rattles me anymore, not since I dealt with multiple surgeries, chemo regimens, and more supplemental treatments than I can even remember. Now, of course, I don't know which one did the trick, but I guess together they worked their magic, because I have been cancer-free for quite some time. In fact, I try to live like that Tim McGraw song, "Live Like You Were Dying," even though I'm not and I would definitely not risk most of the things some other survivors I know have done. The only skydiving I'm doing is from the inside of a large plane on my way to a beach, thank you very much, but I surely appreciate the spirit of that song. Every day I wake up cancer-free, that's a good day and one worth celebrating—on the ground!

Kathy (Indianapolis, Indiana)

Venturing Outside Mainstream Medicine: Complementary, Alternative, and Integrative Options for Managing Side Effects

Once a patient begins investigating other ideas and practices outside the traditional scope of mainstream medicine, she opens up many exciting doors to a variety of healthcare possibilities. Complementary health approaches involve a group of diverse medical and healthcare systems, along with practices and products that originated outside the status quo. These include the use of herbal or other dietary supplements—including medical marijuana—meditation, spinal manipulation, and acupuncture. A worldwide estimate of 33 to 47 percent of people diagnosed with cancer use complementary, alternative, or integrative therapies during their cancer treatment.

Many Americans using these approaches refer to them interchangeably as "alternative" or "complementary," but the terms differ. *Complementary* refers to when a non-mainstream practice is used together with conventional medicine. *Alternative* refers to a nonmainstream practice being used to replace conventional medical techniques.

Integrative joins conventional and complementary approaches in a coordinated way. This idea has continued to grow within healthcare systems across the United States. Researchers are exploring the potential benefits of integrative health in a variety of situations, including pain management for military personnel and veterans, relief of symptoms in cancer patients and survivors, and programs to promote healthy behavior.

Evaluating complementary health care approaches presents challenges. The same careful scientific evaluation that is used to assess conventional therapies should be used to evaluate complementary approaches. Some of these are beginning to find a place in cancer treatment—not as cures, but as additions to treatment plans that may help patients cope with disease symptoms and side effects while improving their overall quality of life.

Although research on the potential value of these integrative programs is in its early stages, some studies have shown promising results. For example, research conducted by the National Center for Complementary and Integrative Health (NCCIH) suggests the following:

- Cancer patients receiving integrative therapies in the hospital have less pain and anxiety.
- Massage therapy may lead to short-term improvements in pain and mood in patients with advanced cancer.
- Yoga may relieve the persistent fatigue some women experience after breast cancer treatment. It's something you can do in a group or alone, and it is well worth investigating.

A substantial amount of scientific evidence suggests that some complementary health approaches may help to manage some symptoms of cancer and side effects of treatment. For other complementary approaches, the evidence is more limited.

There is no convincing evidence at this time that any complementary health approach is effective in curing cancer or causing it to go into remission.

Read the Fine Print!

Unproven products or practices should not be used to replace or delay conventional medical treatment for cancer. Some complementary approaches can interfere with standard cancer treatments or may present special risks for people who have been diagnosed with cancer. Before using any complementary health approach, speak with your healthcare providers to make sure that all aspects of your care work together. Give them a full picture of what you are currently doing to manage your health and a vision of what you would like to try. This will help to ensure coordinated and safe care.

The Society of Integrated Oncology (SIO)[25] is an international organization "dedicated to encouraging scientific evaluation, dissemination of evidence-based information and appropriate clinical integration of complementary therapies." In 2009, they issued evidence-based clinical practice guidelines for healthcare providers to consider when incorporating complementary health approaches in the care of cancer patients. The guidelines point out that, when used in addition to conventional therapies, some of these approaches help to control symptoms and enhance patients' well-being.

SIO recommends[26] that physicians should inquire about the use of complementary and alternative therapies as a routine part of initial evaluations of cancer patients. In addition, all patients with cancer should receive guidance about the advantages and limitations of complementary therapies in an open, evidence-based, and patient-centered manner by a qualified professional. Patients should be fully informed of the treatment approach, the nature of the specific therapies, potential risks/benefits, and realistic expectations.

──────────── MY JOURNEY ────────────

I've always wanted to travel, explore unknown lands, and discover other belief systems. But one should be careful what one wishes for. A few years ago, when I felt something odd under my shoulder and in my breast, I panicked for a second, thinking I had cancer, but I decided not to stress and run to my gynecologist, because I knew a natural healer I really liked. I figured I could just go see him when

────────────

25. *http://integrativeonc.org/*
26. *http://integrativeonc.org/docman-library/uncategorized/65-sio-guidelines-2009/file*

and if I really needed. In the meantime, I began a new, unforeseen trip to the land of denial. A few weeks later, with my chest feeling quite weird, I panicked and contacted my doctor but no appointments were available. I went to see a doctor of Chinese medicine and acupuncture who was also a gynecologist. He did an ultrasound and recommended further testing, which ultimately revealed a malignant tumor.

That day I felt nothing as I walked through my city, watching a movie of the end of my life. Surgery, chemo, radiation: what should I do? I had no idea, but I knew I needed to do something fast. I read everything I could on conventional and experimental treatments. I became a full-time student of every healing technique I could find. A year later, after undergoing every traditional and quack treatment there is, the cancer has returned and I am facing an unknown journey, perhaps to another planet. I have a menu of options to choose from, and no matter which way I go, I know that I must travel deep within myself to get there. The final decision is mine. And I have big plans to go somewhere I have never been before.

Daniela (Santa Cruz, California)

Can Science Support Other Options?

Inside the medical establishment, the debate over complementary, alternative, and integrative treatments continues. Some cancer centers have wholeheartedly embraced a host of these methods and provide them on-site or through off-site partnerships, while other hospitals devoted to cancer care remain skeptical. Regarding insurance companies and what they will pay for, results are mixed and in a steady state of flux. Generally speaking, the jury is still out, but it's clear that trends are moving strongly in the direction of expanding treatment options—not to replace but to support traditional techniques.

So who are we to listen to?

Breast cancer survivor Suzanne Somers, who opted not to do chemotherapy in 2001 after undergoing a lumpectomy and radiation, chose alternative treatments, many of which were controversial at the time and remain so today in certain circles. Her 2009 book, *Knockout: Interviews with Doctors Who Are Curing Cancer—and How to Prevent Getting It in the First Place*, discusses alternate treatments that don't require chemotherapy or radiation, and, in some cases, skip surgery altogether.

Laurie Kirstein, a breast surgical oncologist at Rutgers Cancer Institute of New Jersey in New Brunswick, told *The Asbury Park Press* (NJ) on October 11, 2013, "Suzanne Somers' message may have influenced some people to make dangerous decisions about their treatment without consulting their doctors. Her advice kind of steered women toward just using alternative medicine to treat their breast cancer, and, for most people, will not produce a good result. We promote it, but it should be used alongside medical treatments. When a celebrity comes out with their story, they do have a responsibility to give context and not just promote what they did."

In spite of that, Kirstein and many other professionals in the medical field applaud celebrities for sharing their experiences because it raises cancer awareness and promotes the benefits of early detection, self-breast exams, and the use of mammograms. We agree.

Blending traditional and nontraditional treatments can be a win-win for many people. However, just as patients need to do their due diligence on educating themselves about surgery, chemotherapy, and radiation, they can also gather plenty of available information about the pluses and minuses of complementary, alternative, and integrative options.

For example, substantial evidence exists that acupuncture can help cancer patients manage treatment-related nausea and vomiting. However, there isn't enough evidence yet to judge whether acupuncture relieves cancer pain or other symptoms, such as treatment-related hot flashes. Complications from acupuncture are rare, as long as the acupuncturist uses sterile needles and proper procedures. Chemotherapy and radiation therapy weaken the body's immune system, so it's especially important for acupuncturists to follow strict clean-needle procedures when treating cancer patients.

Studies suggest that the herb ginger may help to control nausea related to cancer chemotherapy when used in addition to conventional antinausea medication. Ginger can be ground up and used to make tea and can also be eaten raw, as you may often see it served with sushi as a palette cleanser.

Studies suggest that massage therapy may help to relieve symptoms experienced by people with cancer, such as pain, nausea, anxiety, and depression. You should consult with your healthcare providers before having massage therapy to find out if any special precautions are needed. For instance, the application of deep or intense pressure is not recommended near cancer lesions or enlarged lymph nodes, radiation field sites, medical devices such as indwelling intravenous catheters (ports), or anatomic distortions such as post-operative changes, or in patients with a bleeding tendency. Since there are many types of massage to choose from—Swedish, shiatsu, Reiki, just to name a few—find out what type of massage may be best for you.

Evidence suggests that mindfulness-based stress reduction, a type of meditation training, can help cancer patients relieve anxiety, stress, fatigue, and general mood and sleep disturbances. Mind-body modalities include yoga, meditation, tai chi, hypnosis, relaxation techniques, and music therapy. You won't know if any of them can help unless you try!

Preliminary evidence indicates that yoga may help to improve anxiety, depression, distress, and stress in people with cancer. It also may help to lessen fatigue in breast cancer patients and survivors. Unfortunately, only a small number of yoga studies in cancer patients have been completed, and the quality of some studies has been questioned. Because yoga involves physical activity, it's important to talk with your healthcare providers in advance to find out whether any aspects of yoga might be unsafe for you. These days, there are many types and levels of yoga practice available in cities and town across America, so it shouldn't be too difficult to find a place that suits your needs.

Various studies suggest possible benefits of hypnosis, relaxation therapies, and biofeedback to help patients manage cancer symptoms and treat side effects.

Therapies based on a philosophy of bioenergy fields (Reiki, therapeutic touch, healing touch, polarity therapy, and external qigong) are safe and may provide some benefit for reducing stress and enhancing a patient's quality of life. There is limited evidence as to their efficacy for symptom management, including reducing pain and fatigue.

Support groups, supportive/expressive therapy, cognitive-behavioral therapy, and cognitive-behavioral stress management are recommended as part of a multidisciplinary approach to reduce anxiety, mood disturbance, chronic pain, and improve quality of life.

More About Supplements

A dietary supplement is a product intended for ingestion that contains a vitamin, mineral, amino acid, herb, or other botanical, enzymes/ingredients intended to add further nutritional value to one's diet. Most claims that refer to the benefits of dietary supplements are anecdotal. In fact, by law, manufacturers are not allowed to claim that their product will cure, treat, or prevent a disease.

Any claim of benefits for some supplements may be supported by early research in a laboratory using cultured cells or lab animals. However, research studies looking for the same benefits in actual patients are very few and usually contain only a few participants.

This makes it difficult to generalize any benefits to a larger patient population.

Studies on whether herbal supplements—or substances derived from them—might be of value in cancer treatment are in their early stages, and scientific evidence is limited. Herbal supplements may have side effects, and some may interact in harmful ways with drugs, including drugs used in cancer treatment.

The effects of taking vitamin and mineral supplements, including antioxidant supplements, during cancer treatment are uncertain. NCI advises cancer patients to talk to their healthcare providers before taking any supplements.

A 2008 review of the research literature on herbal supplements and cancer concluded that although several herbs have shown promise for managing side effects and symptoms, such as nausea and vomiting, pain, fatigue, and insomnia, the scientific evidence is limited, and many clinical trials have not been well designed. Use of herbs for managing symptoms also raises concerns about potential negative interactions with conventional cancer treatments.

In addition, using supplements during chemotherapy or radiation therapy can be problematic because of drug-supplement interactions. For example, some herbs, such as ginkgo, garlic, ginger, bilberry, dong quai, feverfew, ginseng, turmeric, meadowsweet, and willow, contain elements that possess antiplatelet activity. Others, such as chamomile, motherwort, horse chestnut, fenugreek, and red clover, contain coumarin, a chemical used in the synthesis of a number of synthetic blood thinners. Using these while taking anticoagulants (blood thinners) or prior to surgery can increase the risk of bleeding.

Liver toxicity may also be increased by using acetaminophen (Tylenol) along with potentially liver-toxic herbs, echinacea, and kava. Using opioid analgesics along with the sedative herbal supplements, valerian, kava, and chamomile may lead to increased central nervous system (CNS) depression, and ginseng can sometimes inhibit the pain relief effect of opioids.

Patients on tamoxifen or aromatase inhibitors (Chapter 2) should not use red clover, dong quai, or licorice because they contain phytoestrogen (plant estrogen) components. St. John's wort, used by some for depression, can interfere with the metabolism of certain chemotherapy drugs, making them less effective.

These examples point out the importance of honest communications between you and your doctor about any dietary supplements you may be considering. If he or she is not adequately knowledgeable about the use of supplements, then simply ask for a referral to someone in your area who can guide you appropriately.

Olivia Newton-John: East Meets West

Singer and actress Olivia Newton-John was diagnosed with breast cancer in 1992 after finding a small, painful lump. She underwent a partial mastectomy and breast reconstruction followed by chemotherapy. Newton-John also used complementary treatments, such as herbal supplements, acupuncture, meditation, and visualization. "I researched a lot and felt satisfied with my course of treatment. It was sort of an East meets West approach. I meditated every day, did yoga, used homeopathy, ate well—I boosted my inner strength as much as I could. When bad thoughts came in, I pushed them right out."[27]

Buyer Beware

Some products or practices advocated for cancer treatment may interfere with conventional cancer treatments or have other risks. You should consult your healthcare providers before using any

---

27. *http://ww5.komen.org/BreastCancer/OliviaNewtonJohn.html#sthash.WLrKG1i8.dpuf*

complementary health approach. *None of them have cured cancer or caused it to go into remission.*

For example, a 2010 NCCIH-supported trial of a standardized shark cartilage extract, taken in addition to chemotherapy and radiation therapy, showed no benefit in patients with advanced lung cancer. An earlier, smaller study in patients with advanced breast or colorectal cancers also showed no benefit from the addition of shark cartilage to conventional treatment.

A 2011 systematic review of research on laetrile found no evidence that it's effective as a cancer treatment. Laetrile can be toxic, especially if taken orally, because it contains cyanide.

The FDA and the Federal Trade Commission (FTC) have warned the public to be aware of fraudulent cancer treatments. While these scams aren't new, in recent years it has become easier to market them to the public using the Internet.

Some fraudulent cancer treatments are harmful by themselves, and others can be indirectly harmful because people may delay seeking medical care while they try them, or because the fraudulent product interferes with the effectiveness of proven cancer treatments.

Scientific breakthrough!

Get your miraculous cure today!

Secret ingredients to cure you now!

Ancient remedy for today's diseases!

Treats all forms of cancer!

Shrinks malignant tumors instantly!

Recognize any of these advertising pitches? The people who sell fraudulent cancer treatments often market them with claims like these. The advertisements may include personal stories from people who've taken the product, but such stories—real or not—aren't reliable evidence that a product is effective. And a money-back guarantee does not provide proof that a product works.

If you're considering using any anticancer product you've seen in an advertisement, talk to your healthcare provider first. Additional information on cancer-related health frauds is available from the FDA[28] and from the FTC.[29]

Low-Dose Chemotherapy

While traditional chemotherapy is normally prescribed in potent doses, *metronomic* chemotherapy involves the use of lower doses of chemotherapy administered more frequently and regularly, such as weekly or daily. This is in contrast with conventional treatments, which are given at maximum tolerated levels every three weeks at doses just below what have proven to cause over 50 percent of patients to experience severe or dose-limiting toxicity.

Low-dose chemo is intended to ease the burden on a patient, especially when used with naturopathic remedies, which include nutritional and physiological therapies. When combined, these synergistic approaches have been associated with improved treatment consistency, duration, and outcome. These anticancer effects are due to the following elements:

- Anti-angiogenesis
- Improving anti-cancer immune responses by suppressing immune regulatory cells
- Killing more chemo-sensitive cycling cancer cells
- Less tumor cell recovery time between treatments
- Less likelihood of encountering tumor chemo-resistance

Dr. Judah Folkman, former professor at Harvard University and director of the vascular biology program at Children's Hospital Boston,

---

28. *http://www.fda.gov/ForConsumers/ConsumerUpdates/ucm048383.htm*
29. *http://www.ftc.gov/bcp/edu/pubs/consumer/alerts/alt079.pdf*

was the first major proponent of the potential for metronomic chemotherapy in the 1990s, and he inspired many oncologists to explore
these methods.

Nick Chen is a leading medical oncologist and founder of the Seattle
Integrative Cancer Center. According to Ralph W. Moss, PhD, a founding advisor to the National Institute of Health's Office of Alternative
Medicine (now the NCCAM) and advisor to Breast Cancer Action and
the Susan G. Komen Breast Cancer Foundation. "Nick Chen is the
rare medical oncologist who recognizes the importance of nutritional,
mental and emotional health in cancer. When it comes to integrative
oncology," Moss says. "I have seen the future, and it works. As a resi-
dent of a part of the country where naturopathy is not even licensed,
I cast envious eyes on the Pacific Northwest, whose residents have far
greater options when it comes to the varieties of treatment they can
access. I think those who fear the sky will fall if they license naturopathy should study how well it works in states such as Oregon and
Washington, where naturopathy has been accepted since the 1920s."

Dr. Chen presents a persuasive case for giving drugs metronomi-
cally (in low doses) in conjunction with naturopathic post-care, which
he has seen yield remarkable results in certain cancers. Patient results
have also been positive.

Bickley Barich was diagnosed with stage IV metastatic ovarian cancer, and after three years of treatment with heavy chemotherapy, her
oncologist told her there was nothing more he could do. Metronomic
chemotherapy proved to be more effective than her previous treatments, and this integrative approach has given her ten years (and
counting) with her family.

After twelve years with very advanced prostate cancer, Dr. Samuel
Mahaffy is now thriving due in large part to a treatment program
of metronomic chemotherapy in combination with naturopathic
medicine.

We suggest that you investigate these possibilities with your oncologist and see if they are a viable option for you and the particular type of cancer you are treating.

Marijuana and Cancer

Cannabis, also known as marijuana, is a plant that originated in Central Asia and is grown in many parts of the world today, including here in America, although it is still illegal to do so in most parts of the country.

The cannabis plant produces a resin containing compounds called cannabinoids. Some are psychoactive, which act on the brain and change mood or consciousness. In the United States, cannabis is a controlled substance and has been classified as a Schedule I agent (a drug with increased potential for abuse and no known medical use).

Cannabinoids are active chemicals in cannabis that cause drug-like effects throughout the body, including the central nervous system and the immune system. The main active cannabinoid in cannabis is delta-9-THC. Another active cannabinoid is cannabidiol (CBD), which may relieve pain and lower inflammation without causing the "high" of delta-9-THC.

What many people do not know is that our bodies make cannabinoids called endocannabinoids. Many of these are present in the human body; however, the two most common are AEA and 2-AG. Although they may not have the same psychoactive effects as the cannabinoids in marijuana, they still play a key role as a modulator in the functions of neurologic and immune system pathways.

Endocannabinoids exert their effects by binding to specific receptors on their target cells. There are two main types of cannabinoid receptors: CB1 and CB2. CB1 receptors are found mostly in nerve cells (neurons) in the central and peripheral nervous system, while CB2 receptors are most commonly identified in the immune cells.

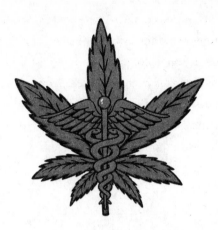

Medical Marijuana
Source: Larry Rains (*istock.com*)

In addition to cannabinoids, marijuana smoke contains many of the same chemical components as tobacco smoke, including arsenic, benzene, formaldehyde, and lead, all of which are known carcinogens. Although it does not contain nicotine, marijuana smoke does contain ammonia, carbon monoxide, hydrogen cyanide, and tar.

Possible effects of cannabinoids include anti-inflammatory activity, antiviral activity, blocking cell growth, preventing the growth of blood vessels that supply tumors, and relieving muscle spasms caused by multiple sclerosis.

Cannabis may be taken by mouth or inhaled. When taken orally (in baked products or as an herbal tea), the main psychoactive ingredient (delta-9-THC) is processed by the liver, which makes an additional psychoactive chemical. Unfortunately, studies of the absorption of THC through the stomach can be slow and erratic, leading to varying amounts in the blood. THC can also be broken down by acid in the stomach.

When cannabis smoke is inhaled, cannabinoids quickly enter the bloodstream. THC is detectable in the blood within seconds and peaks within ten minutes. Another method of inhalation is called vaporization, which uses a device commonly targeted for an e-cigarette. In vaporization, marijuana is heated to a temperature between 180° and 200° C. This releases the active ingredients but only trace amounts of a few other chemicals. It is said to remove approximately 95 percent of the smoke that would otherwise be inhaled.

By federal law, the use, sale, and possession of cannabis (marijuana) is forbidden in the United States. However, a growing number of states (twenty-three at the writing of this book) and the District of Columbia have enacted laws to legalize *medical* marijuana.

Musician Melissa Etheridge used medicinal marijuana during her chemotherapy treatments for breast cancer and says she's continued using it ever since to help cope with the lingering side effects she experienced from the high doses of chemotherapy. In a guest column for CNN, she shared her thoughts on how marijuana helped her. "People use marijuana for different reasons, and I needed it to get me through tough times. I used it every day during chemo: It gave me an appetite so I was able to eat and keep my strength up. It also helped with the depression, and it eased gastrointestinal pain, even to this day. I even find it helps with regulating my sleep."

Pharmaceutical Cannabinoids and the FDA

Two synthetic forms of cannabinoid are approved by the FDA and can be legally prescribed. Dronabinol, available in capsule form, is approved by the FDA to treat chemotherapy-induced nausea and vomiting (CINV) and anorexia associated for weight loss in patients with AIDS.

The second form, nabilone, is approved by the FDA only for CINV. It is also a capsule. The main limitation to both of these drugs is that taking a capsule may be difficult for patients with nausea/vomiting.

One other cannabinol of note is called nabiximols. It is a whole-plant extract of marijuana and contains a ratio of THC to CBD as 1.08:1.00. It is used as an oral mucosal spray and is currently approved for use in Canada and parts of Europe. It is in clinical trials in the United States.

Treating Cancer with Cannabinoids

During laboratory research, cannabinoid receptors have been found on cancer cells and they have been shown to have some antitumor effects.[30] Studies in mice and rats have shown that cannabinoids may inhibit tumor growth by causing cell death, blocking cell growth, and blocking the development of blood vessels needed by tumors to grow. Other animal studies have shown that cannabinoids may kill cancer cells while protecting normal cells.

Clinical trials in patients, however, have been extremely limited. For this reason, there are no current recommendations for the use of marijuana in the direct treatment of cancer.

Tommy Chong Uses Marijuana to Treat His Cancers

Canadian comedian, actor, writer, director, activist, and former *Dancing with the Stars* contestant Tommy Chong told *US Weekly* in June 2015 that he had been diagnosed with rectal cancer. In true Cheech and Chong fashion, he tweeted: "I have good news and bad news. First the bad news, the cancer came back and it's a real pain in the butt."

In an interview with *Access Hollywood Live*, Chong said that he sought medical advice when he began to experience blood in his stool and was told that his cancer was in stage I. He said he would undergo

---

30. Joan L. Kramer, MD, CA, "Medical Marijuana for Cancer, *A Cancer Journal for Clinicians*, vol. 65, no. 2, Mar/Apr 2015: 109–122.

a short course of chemotherapy and radiation therapy before having the tumor removed surgically, which he did in October 2015.

This is not Chong's first time dealing with cancer. Three years earlier, he was diagnosed with cancer of the prostate. As a vocal marijuana-legalization advocate, Chong used cannabis oil (as a suppository) to treat his cancer and smoked marijuana to relieve some of his symptoms. "I'm using cannabis like crazy now," he told *US Weekly* at the time. "More so than ever before. I'm in treatment now, and either I get healed or I don't. But either way, I'm going to make sure I get a little edge off or put up."

Using Medical Marijuana to Treat Side Effects

While its potential to treat cancer as a disease is yet to be determined, medical marijuana has already proven to be beneficial for many cancer patients in treating some of the side effects of treatment:

- Chemotherapy-induced nausea and vomiting (CINV)
- Poor appetite and weight loss
- Pain
- Anxiety
- Sleep deprivation

Despite advances in pharmacologic and nonpharmacological management, nausea and vomiting remain distressing side effects for cancer patients and their families. As previously mentioned, both dronabinol and nabilone are now approved by the FDA for the treatment of chemotherapy-induced nausea and vomiting.

Let's look at how medical marijuana might treat some side effects of cancer treatments, as well as some side effects of cannabinoids.

Chemotherapy-Induced Nausea and Vomiting (CINV)

There are also several studies looking at smoked marijuana and CINV. In one review of over 1,300 patients, cannabinoids were found to be more effective than conventional antiemetics, such as prochlorperazine, metoclopramide, chlorpromazine, thiethylperazine, haloperidol, domperidone, and alizapride. However, reported side effects included a feeling of being high, euphoria, sedation or drowsiness, dizziness, dysphoria or depression, hallucinations, paranoia, and hypotension (low blood pressure).

Poor Appetite and Weight Loss

Anorexia, early satiety, weight loss, and cachexia are common problems for cancer patients. Some are faced not only with the disfigurement associated with these symptoms but also with the inability to engage in the social interaction of meals.

Perhaps not surprisingly, trials conducted in the 1980s that involved healthy control subjects showed that inhaling *marijuana* led to an increase in caloric intake, mainly in the form of between-meal snacks, with increased intakes of fatty and sweet foods. The question is, would this effect also be seen in cancer patients?

Three controlled trials demonstrated that oral THC has variable effects on appetite stimulation and weight loss in patients with advanced malignancies and human immunodeficiency virus (HIV) infection. Some studies showed increased appetite, but weight gain did not necessarily accompany the improvement in appetite. One study showed that dronabinol could improve altered taste sensations associated with chemotherapy.

Pain

Cancer pain results from inflammation, invasion of bone or other pain-sensitive structures, or nerve injury. When cancer pain is severe and persistent, it is often resistant to treatment with opioids. Managing or, in some cases, even relieving pain, which medical marijuana has been shown to do, improves a patient's quality of life through all stages of cancer.

Two studies examined the effects of oral delta-9-THC on cancer pain. The first, a double-blind placebo-controlled study involving ten patients, measured both pain intensity and pain relief.[31] It was reported that 15 mg and 20 mg doses of the cannabinoid delta-9-THC were associated with substantial analgesic effects, with antiemetic effects and appetite stimulation.

Another study[32] examined the effects of a plant extract with controlled cannabinoid content in an oromucosal spray. In a multicenter, double-blind, placebo-controlled study, the THC:CBD nabiximols extract and THC extract alone were compared in the analgesic management of patients with advanced cancer and with moderate-to-severe cancer-related pain. The researchers concluded that the THC:CBD extract was efficacious for pain relief in advanced cancer patients whose pain was not fully relieved by strong opioids.

Anxiety

A small number of studies have shown that the use of cannabinoid delta-9-THC is associated with a reduction in a patient's anxiety. Depending on their previous experience, patients often experience mood elevation after exposure to cannabis. In a five-patient case series of inhaled cannabis that examined analgesic effects in chronic pain, it was reported that patients who self-administered cannabis had improved mood and sense of well-being, and less anxiety.

---

31. http://www.ncbi.nlm.nih.gov/pubmed/1091664?dopt=Abstract

32. http://www.ncbi.nlm.nih.gov/pubmed/19896326?dopt=Abstract

Sleep Deprivation

One small placebo-controlled study of dronabinol in cancer patients noted an increased quality of sleep and relaxation in those treated with THC. Another common effect of cannabis is sleepiness. A small placebo-controlled study of dronabinol in cancer patients with altered chemosensory perception also noted an increased quality of sleep and relaxation in those treated with THC.

The Flip Side: Adverse Effects

Because cannabinoid receptors, unlike opioid receptors, are not located in the brainstem areas controlling respiration, lethal overdoses from cannabis and cannabinoids do *not* occur. However, cannabinoid receptors are present in other tissues throughout the body, not just in the central nervous system, and adverse effects include rapid heartbeat, low blood pressure, red eyes, muscle relaxation, and slowed gastrointestinal motility.

Although cannabinoids are considered by some to be addictive drugs, their addictive potential is considerably lower than that of other prescribed agents or substances of abuse. The brain, however, can develop a tolerance to cannabinoids.

Withdrawal symptoms such as irritability, insomnia with sleep electroencephalogram disturbance, restlessness, hot flashes, and, rarely, nausea and cramping have been observed. However, these symptoms appear to be mild compared with withdrawal symptoms associated with opiates or benzodiazepines, and the symptoms usually dissipate after a few days.

Since cannabis smoke contains many of the same components as tobacco smoke, there are valid concerns about the adverse pulmonary effects of inhaled cannabis. Marijuana smoke can cause injury to the lungs and airways, but there is no clear link to marijuana smoke and the development of chronic obstructive pulmonary disease (COPD). Many of the effects of marijuana smoke subside after marijuana use has stopped.

> **NOTE to PATIENT:**
> For more information, visit *www.reimaginingcancer.com.*

Bringing Mind and Body Together

Cancer centers throughout the country are discovering that providing genuine, lasting wellness for their patients may require more than the traditional methods they have offered in the past. As a result, they are incorporating a menu of new options that complement and expand existing methods of treatment. These new offerings generally focus on the multiple benefits of connecting the mind and body—as a tool to combat side effects, as a method for better communication between patients and doctors, and as a viable means for patients to express and process the many levels of vulnerability that any diagnosis of cancer creates.

For example, patient services in many cancer centers now offer art therapy that may include painting and sculpture classes, dance, theater, and writing programs. Each of these has proven to be remarkable opportunities for patients (and caregivers) to relieve stress while providing outlets for much-needed personal expression.

Writing, in particular, seems to offer multiple possibilities for patients to explore their feelings as well as to document their experience for pragmatic purposes.

According to Nancy Morgan, a writing clinician and director of the Arts and Humanities program at Lombardi Comprehensive Cancer Center at Georgetown University in Washington, DC, "Twenty years of research in controlled laboratory settings indicates writing may contribute to improved physical and emotional health . . . we found that just one writing session in a busy cancer clinic where the patients are frequently interrupted can still have a positive impact on patients."[33]

Morgan's studies suggest a strong possibility that writing down thoughts and feelings can change a patient's view of her cancer, opening up another door to improving her quality of life, even from a physical perspective.

Many patients reported that, although they don't necessarily like talking about cancer, writing about it certainly helped them get through it.[34]

Bruce D. Cheson, MD, head of hematology at Lombardi and a coauthor on the study, reported, "Many of our patients were interested in this kind of therapy. Our study supports the benefit of an expressive writing program and the ability to integrate such a program into a busy clinic."

What If?

What if you began expressing yourself in writing and that led you to communicate more effectively with your family, friends, and doctors? What if writing relieved some of your stress and helped you feel more in control of your situation? What if other people in your life became inspired by how you began coping with your challenges?

"Who am I?" touches us on spiritual and pragmatic levels. It can be both an existential and a moment-by-moment question. In times of great change and stress, such as in response to a diagnosis of cancer, our sense of self will be questioned, and the ways in which we previously identified ourselves may be turned upside down. Whether

---

33. *The Oncologist*, February 2008.
34. *Coping with Cancer*, March/April 2009.

you are a patient or a caregiver of any kind, it's vital that you see life with clear eyes, and that begins each morning when you look in the mirror. If you've been diagnosed with cancer, you're probably facing enormous challenges and need to focus a great deal on yourself. If you are a patient's caretaker, doctor, or nurse—responsible for someone else's health—you also need to take care of yourself. Writing can help. You can begin with two simple exercises and *no* rules. You're the boss of you, not your high school English teacher.

The first is called, "I AM" and asks you to listen to the core of your mind and body. Start with those two words—I AM—and just write whatever comes to mind. It may be emotional or philosophical or physical or all three somehow combined. There are no wrong answers! But there are compelling reasons for getting in touch with yourself, especially when your very existence is being challenged.

The second exercise involves writing a simple "To Do" list. If you or someone you care about has been diagnosed with cancer, that list has suddenly been expanded with an entire new set of protocols to handle, from keeping track of doctors' appointments and medication regimens to communicating with family, friends, and colleagues about how cancer—directly or indirectly—is affecting your life. That can be daunting, so do yourself a favor and get organized. Write down what you need to do and when, who you want to talk to and how you wish to approach them. Each To Do on the list is bound to beg for more. But more is good. It means you're getting things done, including the challenging tasks you may ordinarily avoid.

Let your list encourage you to live in the moment and guide you with courage into an uncertain future. Take a few minutes to write down the small things, and while you're at it take a stab at the big issues, too. Surprises are waiting with each step you take.[35]

---

35. From David Tabatsky, *Write for Life: Communicating Your Way Through Cancer* (2013).

And While You're At It—the Healing Power of Laughter

If you could bottle laughter and offer it for sale, pharmacies all over the world would be selling it like hotcakes and turning into palaces. After all, what feels better than laughing?

We've all heard the saying, "Laughter is the best medicine." We've also heard endless claims from shamans, traveling salesmen, and websites about holistic, organic cures for everything under the sun. As far as we know, only three things exist that contain the therapeutic qualities needed to cure anything: love, positivity, and laughter. Without these three, even the strongest medicine may not do the trick.

When things are bad; when the fear is great and the treatments are harsh; when you're puking all night and your hair falls out; when your wife goes bald or your husband goes limp; when your patience fails or you just don't know what to do, how in God's name are you to survive—even for another day?

Laughter. We were born with this gift. It can elevate our spirits and make us happy. Laughter is contagious, too. It brings people together. If you get on a good roll, you'll feel stronger and more alive, no matter what shape you're in or how bad you feel.

Norman Cousins, a former editor at the *Saturday Review*, put the concept of laugh therapy on the map in 1976 when his article in the *New England Journal of Medicine* described how he had been afflicted with a rare degenerative disease of the connective tissue. After suffering a series of setbacks in the hospital, he decided to check into a hotel, take massive doses of vitamin C, watch Marx Brothers movies, and read funny books for days on end. Eventually, his symptoms abated and most of the freedom of movement he had lost he eventually regained. Cousins beautifully told his story of the power of the mind on the body in his book *Anatomy of an Illness* (Norton, 1979). Although no one in the medical community can say for sure what

essentially cured Cousins, his story does seem to suggest that love, positivity, and laughter can be effective allies in the fight against disease.

───────────────── **MY JOURNEY** ─────────────────

Over a span of several years, my husband was diagnosed four separate times with cancer. It became fairly normal to hear people's shock
when they heard his story. They were usually tongue-tied, especially
when he told them, "I'm trying out a few different cancers and I hope
I find one I really like." It was amazing to see people's reactions, and
it does suggest that cancer is something we can actually live with—
maybe even "live long and prosper."

Melanie (Roanoke, Virginia)

How do you have fun? What makes you laugh? Can you describe
three things that make you laugh? Of course, no one will stop you if
you don't stop at three and keep going—that is definitely encouraged.

For people living with cancer, it may seem strange or even distaste-
ful to consider humor when facing such serious issues. Yet, laughter can be helpful in ways you might not have realized or imagined.
Laughter can help you feel better about yourself and the world around
you. Have you looked at the world lately? It's pretty funny. Then again,
it's pretty sad, and we need comic relief—lots of it.

Laughter is a natural diversion. When you laugh, no other thought
comes to mind. Laughing can also induce physical changes in the
body. After laughing for just a few minutes, you may feel better for
hours. When used to supplement conventional cancer treatments,
laughter therapy may help in the overall healing process. According
to some studies, laughter therapy may provide physical benefits, such
as boosting the immune system and circulatory system; enhancing

oxygen intake; stimulating the heart and lungs; relaxing muscles throughout the body; triggering the release of endorphins (the body's natural painkillers); easing digestion; soothing stomachaches; relieving pain; balancing blood pressure; and improving mental functions (i.e., alertness, memory, creativity).

Laughter therapy may also improve overall attitude, reduce stress and tension, promote relaxation, aid sleep, enhance quality of life, strengthen social bonds and relationships, and produce a general sense of well-being.

In fact, some cancer centers have started support groups dedicated to creating laughter as part of their mind-body wellness programs. It's a form of physical and emotional therapy that helps patients cope while receiving conventional cancer treatments. According to many participants, they were able to leave their troubles at the door and stop thinking about cancer. Instead, they learned that even while dealing with what sometimes may feel like an insurmountable challenge, they come to realize that they *can* still laugh and even feel better.

Sounds like just what the doctor ordered.[36]

---

36. From David Tabatsky, *Write for Life: Communicating Your Way Through Cancer* (2013).

KEY POINTS TO REMEMBER

✓ Save your energy and balance rest with activity.

✓ Eat and drink well, and seek nutritional counseling.

✓ Use medicines and treatments prescribed by your doctor.

✓ Palliative care is not specifically end-of-life care. It offers you a plan to manage pain and can be quite temporary.

✓ Wash your hands often and well.

✓ Avoid foods that are greasy, fried, sweet, or spicy, and eat a small snack before treatment.

✓ Ask about pain medicine and integrative medicine practices.

✓ Keep track of your pain profile.

✓ Take pain medicine as prescribed.

✓ Tell your doctor about problems that interfere with sleep, and set good bedtime habits.

✓ Cancer patients receiving integrative therapies in the hospital have less pain and anxiety.

✓ Massage therapy may lead to short-term improvements in pain and mood in patients with advanced cancer.

✓ Yoga may relieve persistent fatigue that some women experience after breast cancer treatment.

✓ Read the fine print! If you're considering using any anticancer product you've seen in an advertisement, talk to your healthcare provider first.

✓ Medical marijuana has proven to be beneficial for many cancer patients in treating some of the side effects of treatment.

That Kind of Love

My mom has no breasts.

Uterus? Bye-bye.

Ovaries? Gone.

Fallopian tubes? Ha.

If I look at her skin, it starts to itch.

If she throws up any more, she may disappear.

Her hair fell out during dinner one night
and no one cried into their soup.
We swept it up and kept eating.

Cancer? Ugh.

My mom is a leftover,
but my dad still loves her.

Yep.
That's the kind of love I want when I grow up.

—Miriam Hamilton

13

SAVE YOUR OWN LIFE: How to Prevent Cancer or Catch It Early

The only thing we have to fear is fear itself.
So the only thing to really be afraid of is if
you don't go get your mammograms.
Because there's some part of you
that doesn't want to know,
and that's the thing that's going to trip you up.
That's the thing that could have
a really bad endgame.

—**Cynthia Nixon**, as told to *abcnews.go.com*

Bad Luck or Bad Environment?

In January 2015, renowned cancer researcher Bert Vogelstein of Johns Hopkins University School of Medicine published a study suggesting that developing certain types of cancer is just the result of "bad luck." Some people in the field interpreted his work to mean that screening and early detection might be more important than preventing cancer from developing in the first place. This spin on Dr. Vogelstein's data was so controversial that it created a firestorm of clashing views about how much time, effort, and money we should spend trying to prevent the disease if, indeed, developing cancer is mostly the result of bad luck.

One year later, in January 2016, a group of researchers from Stony Brook University published a study that came to the opposite conclusion, declaring that most cancers are caused by factors in our environments and can therefore be prevented. Here's the Stony Brook list of preventable cancers and the factors that cause them.

Cancer Type	Preventable Risk	Risk Factors
Anus	>63%	HPV infection, smoking
Breast	Substantial	Oral contraceptives, hormone replacement therapy, lifestyle factors (diet & weight, smoking & drinking)
Cervix	~90%	HPV infection
Colon & rectum	>75%	Diet, smoking, alcohol, obesity
Esophagus	>75%	Smoking, alcohol, obesity, diet
Head & neck	>75%	Tobacco & alcohol
Kidney	>58%	Smoking, obesity, workplace exposures
Liver	~80%	Hepatitis B and C virus infections
Lung	>90%	Smoking, air pollution
Lymphoma	>71%	Chemicals, radiation, immune system deficiency
Mouth & voice box	~70%	HPV infection

Prostate	Substantial	Diet, smoking, obesity
Skin—melanoma	65–86%	Sun exposure
Skin—basal cell	~90%	Ultraviolet (UV) radiation
Stomach	65–80%	Helicobacter pylori infection
Thyroid	>72%	Diet low in iodine, radiation

So who's right, Dr. Vogelstein or the Stony Brook scientists?

They both are.

At its root, cancer is a disease of your DNA. You inherit your DNA from your parents, and it really is a matter of luck which combinations of genes you end up with. If some of these genes can cause cancer or just make you more likely to develop certain types (as described in Chapter 3), knowing your family medical history, screening, and early detection will be the main tools for saving your life.

However, most cancers are not caused by inherited genes but by damage to your DNA that occurs in your lifetime. As the Stony Brook researchers pointed out, depending on the type of cancer, we can reduce our risk of developing cancer by 60 to 90 percent through changes in our lifestyles and environment.

Environment and Lifestyle Factors

For many years, researchers have been studying several ways to help prevent cancer. Considering some factors, the evidence is conclusive; while for others, things are not so clear. The following table shows some of the risk factors/exposures that possess ample evidence linking them to cancer.

Risk Factor	Examples	Preventable Cancers
Cigarette smoking and tobacco	Cigarettes, smokeless tobacco	Acute myelogenous leukemia (AML) Bladder Esophagus Kidney Lung Mouth and tongue Pancreas Stomach
Infections	HPV Hepatitis B and C Epstein Barr Virus Helicobacter pylori HIV-AIDS	Cervix, penis, vagina, anus, oral Liver Burkitt's lymphoma Stomach Kaposi sarcoma
Radiation	UV radiation Ionizing radiation	Skin cancers Leukemia, thyroid, breast
Drugs that suppress the immune system	Transplant patients	Non-Hodgkin lymphoma (NHL), lung, kidney, liver

A number of factors may affect the risk of cancer, but the overall evidence among them is not as strong. These factors include diet, alcohol, physical activity, obesity, and diabetes. It is hard to study the effects of diet on cancer because your diet may include both foods that protect against cancer as well as foods that may increase the risk of cancer. It is also hard for participants in studies to keep track of what they eat over a long period of time. This may be one explanation why studies looking at the effect of diet on cancer risk can have different results.

Other lifestyle factors are also hard to study. It is common knowledge that people who are physically active have a lower risk of certain cancers than those who are not, but it is not known if physical activity itself is the reason for this. And although it is known that those with obesity have a higher rate of cancer, we don't know whether losing weight decreases that risk.

The role of diabetes in cancer is further complicated by the fact that many of the risk factors that cause diabetes (diet, obesity, lack of activity, and smoking) also affect one's cancer risk. It is hard to know whether the risk of cancer is increased more by diabetes or by these risk factors themselves. Studies are underway to see how medicine that is used to treat diabetes affects cancer risk.

This table outlines these factors that *may* affect the risk of cancer. Arrows pointing up indicate a possible increased risk, while arrows pointing down indicate the possibility of a decreased risk.

Risk Factor	↑/↓	Cancer
Diet		
Fruit and non-starchy vegetables	↓	Oral cancer
		Esophageal cancer
		Stomach cancer
Fruit	↓	Lung cancer
Diet high in fat, protein, red meat	↑/↓	Colorectal cancer
Low fat, high fiber, high fruits and vegetables.	↓	Colorectal cancer
Alcohol	↑	Oral cancer
	↑	Esophageal cancer
	↑	Breast cancer
	↑	Colorectal cancer (in men)
	↑	Liver and colorectal cancer (in women)

Physical activity	⬇	Colorectal cancer
	⬇	Postmenopausal breast cancer
	⬇	Endometrial cancer
Obesity	⬆	Postmenopausal breast cancer
	⬆	Colorectal cancer
	⬆	Endometrial cancer
	⬆	Esophageal cancer
	⬆	Kidney cancer
	⬆	Pancreatic cancer
	⬆	Cancer of the gallbladder
Diabetes	⬆	Bladder cancer
	⬆	Breast cancer in women
	⬆	Colorectal cancer
	⬆	Endometrial cancer
	⬆	Liver cancer
	⬆	Lung cancer
	⬆	Oral cancer
	⬆	Oropharyngeal cancer
	⬆	Ovarian cancer
	⬆	Pancreatic cancer
Environmental Risk Factors		
Air pollution, secondhand smoke, asbestos	⬆	Lung cancer
Arsenic in drinking water	⬆	Skin cancer
	⬆	Bladder cancer
	⬆	Lung cancer

Factors Suspected to Affect Cancer Risk. Source: *CelebrityDiagnosis.com*

But I Did Everything Right!

For some women with cancer, the shock of the diagnosis is often accompanied with bewilderment that this could have happened to someone who faithfully followed the rules of healthy living. Gill Deacon, one of Canada's best-known environmental writers and a virtual poster child for mindful living and sustainable consumption, is one of those people. She was diagnosed with breast cancer at the age of forty-two, and it came as a slap in the face to someone who, according to her, "measured carbon emissions, rode her bike in the rain, said no to high fructose corn syrup and yes to rabbit food."

In her memoir *Naked Imperfection* (Penguin Canada, 2014), Gill writes about her breast cancer experience and how she came to realize that her "lifestyle wasn't an antidote to misfortune."

Gill's story is one of an overachiever who had lived her whole life trying to maintain control and attain various ideals of perfection. She approached breast cancer as "the newest challenge to be met, survival just one more thing to achieve." Gill eventually came to the realization that cancer is not just something else she can control and that the outcome is not entirely in her hands. Fortunately, her outcome has been positive and she now regards cancer as a gift—albeit one wrapped in barbed wire—that has given her a new perspective on life.

Chemoprevention

Chemoprevention refers to the use of substances to lower the risk of cancer or keep it from recurring. The substances may be natural or made in a laboratory. Some chemopreventive agents are tested in people who are at high risk for a certain type of cancer. The risk may be because of a precancerous condition, family history, or lifestyle factors.

Some chemoprevention studies have shown good results. Treatment with tamoxifen lowers the risk of estrogen receptor-positive (ER-positive) breast cancer and DCIS (Chapter 2) in premenopausal and postmenopausal women at high risk. Treatment with raloxifene also lowers the risk of breast cancer in postmenopausal women. With either drug, the reduced risk lasts for several years or longer after treatment is stopped. Lower rates of broken bones have been noted in patients taking raloxifene.

Aromatase inhibitors (anastrozole, letrozole) and inactivators (exemestane), which decrease the amount of estrogen made by the body, lower the risk of a new breast cancer in women who have a history of breast cancer. Aromatase inhibitors also decrease the risk of breast cancer in postmenopausal women with a personal history of breast cancer, women with no personal history of breast cancer who are sixty years and older, women who have a history of DCIS with mastectomy, or women who have a high risk of cancer based on their answers to the National Cancer Institute's Breast Cancer Risk Assessment Tool *(http://www.cancer.gov/bcrisktool/)*.

Chemoprevention agents that are being studied to prevent breast and colorectal cancers include inhibitors of an enzyme called COX-2, which block the production of prostaglandins that promote inflammation. Although evidence suggests that COX-2 inhibitors can prevent colon and breast cancer, their usefulness may be limited by an increased risk of cardiovascular side effects, such as stroke.

Aspirin is being studied for the prevention of invasive ovarian cancer and breast cancer, as well as for colorectal cancer.

Contrary to popular claims, there is currently not enough scientific evidence to show that vitamin and dietary supplements prevent cancer. Several vitamins and minerals have been studied, including vitamin B6, vitamin B12, vitamin E, vitamin D, beta carotene, folic acid, and selenium, but they have not been shown to lower the risk of cancer.

> **NOTE to PATIENT:**
> Learn about your family medical history!
> As discussed in Chapters 3 and 6,
> it is one of the most important risk factors for many cancers.
> Consider making a pedigree diagram (Chapter 3)
> of your family to share with your doctor.

HPV Vaccine: A Poster Child for Cancer Prevention

Armed with the knowledge that human papillomavirus (HPV) is the cause of a number of cancers, including cervical, vaginal, anal, and head and neck cancers, researchers have been able to move on to the next logical step. By creating a vaccine, which would prevent the infection in people exposed to it, they hoped to decrease or eliminate the risk of HPV leading to cancer.

Cancer vaccines belong to a class of substances known as biological response modifiers. These work by stimulating or restoring the immune system's ability to fight infections and disease. There are two broad types of cancer vaccines:

1. Preventive (prophylactic) vaccines intend to prevent cancer from developing in healthy people.
2. Treatment (therapeutic) vaccines intend to treat an existing cancer by strengthening the body's natural immune response against the cancer. Treatment vaccines are a form of immunotherapy.

Two types of cancer preventive vaccines (human papillomavirus vaccines and hepatitis B virus vaccines) are available in the United States, and one treatment vaccine (for metastatic prostate cancer) is also available.

How Cancer-Preventative Vaccines Work

Cancer-preventive vaccines target infectious agents that cause or contribute to the development of cancer. They are similar to traditional vaccines, which help prevent infectious diseases, such as measles or polio, by protecting the body against infection. Both cancer preventive vaccines and traditional vaccines are based on antigens (markers) found on the infectious agents, which the immune system recognizes as foreign. Preventive vaccines stimulate the production of antibodies that bind to specific targeted microbes and block their ability to cause infection.

Cancer preventive vaccines approved by the FDA to date have been made using antigens from Hepatitis B (HBV, one cause of liver cancer) and specific types of HPV. These antigens are proteins that help make up the outer surface of the viruses. Because only part of these microbes is used, the resulting vaccines are not infectious and, therefore, cannot cause disease.

Similarly, cancer treatment vaccines are made using cancer-associated antigens or modified versions of them. Antigens that have been used thus far include proteins, carbohydrates (sugars), glyco-proteins or glycopeptides (carbohydrate-protein combinations), and gangliosides (carbohydrate-lipid combinations).

Before any vaccine is licensed, the FDA must conclude that it is both safe and effective. Vaccines intended to prevent or treat cancer appear to have safety profiles comparable to those of other vaccines. However, the side effects of cancer vaccines can vary among vaccine formulations—and from one person to another.

The most commonly reported side effect of cancer vaccines is inflammation at the site of injection, along with a chance of redness, pain, warming of the skin, itchiness, and even a rash.

People sometimes experience flu-like symptoms after receiving a cancer vaccine, including fever, chills, weakness, dizziness, nausea or vomiting, muscle ache, fatigue, headache, and occasional breathing difficulties. Blood pressure may also be affected. These side effects, which usually last for only a short time, indicate that the body is responding to the vaccine and making an immune response as it does when exposed to a virus.

For more information about the HPV vaccine, see Chapter 8.

Cancer Screening: A Harm/Benefit Analysis

Checking for cancer—or conditions that may become cancer—in people who have no symptoms is called screening. It can help doctors find and treat several types of cancer before they become more difficult to treat. Early detection is important because when abnormal tissue or cancer is found early, it may be easier to treat. By the time symptoms appear, cancer may have begun to spread and is harder to treat. Several screening tests have been shown to detect cancer early and to reduce the chance of dying from that cancer.

But it is important to note the potential risks when it comes to screening tests because they can present potential harmful effects along with their benefits. Some of these include the following:

- *Bleeding* or other health problems may occur as a result of a screening process.
- *False-positive results* indicate that cancer may be present, even though it is not. False-positive test results can cause anxiety and are usually followed by additional tests and procedures that also may be harmful.
- *False-negative results* indicate that cancer is *not* present, even though it is. These test results may provide incorrect reassurance, delaying a proper diagnosis, and may cause an individual to put off seeking medical care even if symptoms develop.

- *Overdiagnosis* is possible when a screening test correctly shows
  that a person has cancer, but the cancer is slow growing and
  would not have harmed that person in his or her lifetime.
  Treatment of such cancers is called overtreatment.

Breast Cancer and Mammograms

As we first described in Chapter 2, a mammogram is an X-ray image of the breast. It can be used as a tool to screen for breast cancer in women who have no signs or symptoms of the disease. Screening mammograms usually involve two X-ray images of each breast. These images make it possible to detect tumors that are not large enough to be felt by the woman or her doctor. Screening mammograms can also find micro-calcifications (tiny deposits of calcium) that sometimes indicate the presence of breast cancer.

Mammograms can also be used to check for breast cancer after a lump or other sign or symptom of the disease has been found. This type of mammogram is called a diagnostic mammogram, which can also be used to evaluate changes found during a screening mammogram, or to view breast tissue when it is difficult to obtain a screening mammogram because of special circumstances, such as the presence of breast implants.

Mammograms: When and How Often?

There is no doubt that mammography has saved lives. In the randomized controlled trials (RCTs), for women aged forty to seventy-four years, screening with mammography has been associated with a 15 to 20 percent relative reduction in mortality from breast cancer.

As discussed in Chapter 2, three organizations make recommendations on the age and frequency for women to undergo screening mammograms: The American Cancer Society (ACS), The American College of Obstetricians and Gynecologists (ACOG), and the U.S.

Preventive Services Task Force (USPSTF). Unfortunately, the three organizations each have their own guidelines, which can lead to confusion among women and their doctors.

In October 2015, the ACS revised their mammography guidelines. The changes included three main points:

1. Begin regular screening at forty-five instead of at forty years. Women between forty and forty-five should have the option of screening.
2. Women fifty-five years and older should transition to every-other-year mammography but should still have the option to have them annually.
3. Clinical breast examinations are no longer recommended for breast cancer screening.

Shortly thereafter, in January 2016, the USPSTF released their newest guideline recommendations. They recommended a mammogram every two years for women fifty to seventy-four years of age and considered it an individualized decision to screen between forty and forty-nine. They recommended against teaching breast self-exams because this practice has no clear net benefit.

In response to the revised ACS recommendations, ACOG released a statement in October 2015: "ACOG strongly supports shared decision making between doctor and patient, and in the case of screening for breast cancer, it is essential. We recognize that guidelines and recommendations evolve as new evidence emerges, but currently ACOG continues to support routine mammograms beginning at forty years as well as continued use of clinical breast examinations."[37]

This chart summarizes the recommendation guidelines of the three organizations.

---

37. *http://www.acog.org/About-ACOG/News-Room/Statements/2015/ACOG-Statement-on-Recom mendations-on-Breast-Cancer-Screening*

Population	ACS 2015	USPSTF	ACOG
Women aged 40–44	Women should have the opportunity to begin annual screening between the ages of 40–44	The decision to start regular, biennial screening mammography before 50 should be an individual one and take patient context into account including the patient's values regarding specific benefits and harms	Screening mammograms every year for women aged 40–49
Women aged 45–54	Women should undergo regular screening mammography beginning at 45. Women 45–54 should be screened annually.	The USPSTF concludes that the current evidence is insufficient to assess the additional benefits and harms of clinical breast examination beyond screening mammography in women 40 years or older.	Screening mammograms every year for women aged 50 or older.
Women ≥ 55	Women 55 and older should transition to biennial screening or have the opportunity to continue screening annually. Women should continue screening mammography as long as their overall health is good and they have a life expectancy of 10 years or longer.	The USPSTF recommends biennial screening mammography for women 50–74. The USPSTF concludes that the current evidence is insufficient to assess the benefits and harms of the screening mammography in women 75 and older.	Screening mammograms every year for women 55 and older.
All women	Clinical breast examination is not recommended for breast cancer screening among average-risk women at any age. All women should become familiar with the potential benefits, limitations, and harms associated with breast cancer screening.	The USPSTF recommends against teaching breast self-examination (BSE). The USPSTF concludes that the current evidence is insufficient to assess the additional benefits and harms of either digital mammography or magnetic resonance imaging (MRI) instead of film mammography as screening modalities for breast cancer.	Clinical breast exam every year for women 19 and older.

It's important to realize that these recommendations are based on statistics that apply to "average" women in the United States. But not every woman has average risks, and only you and your primary care doctor, informed by your current health and family medical history, can determine what choices are right for you.

Potential Risks of Screening Mammograms

Finding cancer does not always mean saving lives. Although mammograms can detect malignant tumors that cannot be felt during an external breast exam, treating a small tumor does not always mean that a woman's life will be saved. In spite of detecting a tumor, a fast-growing or aggressive cancer may have already spread to other parts of the body before it is detected.

Screening mammograms can find a condition called ductal carcinoma *in situ* (DCIS) (sometimes referred to as stage 0 breast cancer), which signifies a noninvasive lesion where abnormal cells form in the lining of breast ducts. (See section on DCIS in Chapter 2.)

Mammograms require very small doses of radiation. The risk of harm from this exposure is low, but repeated X-rays have the potential to cause cancer. The benefits, however, nearly always outweigh the risks. A woman receiving any type of X-ray should think about whether she might be pregnant. If she has any doubt at all, she should alert her doctor and the mammography technician.

Just as with any screening test, mammograms can also yield undesirable and misleading information, false-negative results, false-positive results, and/or overdiagnosis and overtreatment. False-negative results occur when mammograms appear normal, even though breast cancer is present, leading to delays in treatment and a false sense of security for affected women. False-positive results can happen when radiologists decide mammograms are abnormal but no cancer is actually present. This is more common among younger women, those who have had previous breast biopsies, women with a family history of breast cancer, and individuals taking estrogen (for example, to alleviate menopause). False-positive mammogram results can lead to anxiety and other forms of psychological distress in affected women.

Any additional testing required to rule out cancer can be costly, time-consuming, and a source of physical discomfort. However, please take note that *all* abnormal mammograms should be followed up with additional testing (diagnostic mammograms, ultrasound, and/ or biopsy) to determine whether cancer is present.

Sheryl Crow: Making Better Decisions

The year 2005 seemed like a good year for singer, songwriter, and actress Sheryl Crow. She became engaged to Tour de France bicyclist Lance Armstrong, released her fifth studio album, *Wildflower*, and was nominated for a Grammy for Best Female Pop Vocal Performance for her hit single "Good Is Good."

But things took a dramatic term by the beginning of 2006. Just six days after announcing that she and Lance had ended their engagement, her doctor reported that her routine mammogram showed suspicious calcifications in both breasts. Sheryl was ultimately diagnosed with ductal carcinoma *in situ* and underwent an immediate lumpectomy followed by seven weeks of radiation and supplemented with acupuncture, herbal tea, and meditation, which she began practicing to help her relax and to give her body the chance to function at a higher cellular level,[38] which it tends to do when relaxed. Because the disease was caught early, she did not have to undergo chemotherapy.

"I am a walking advertisement for early detection," Sheryl Crow told *AARP The Magazine* in October 2006. "I recommend regular mammograms, and if I knew I had the BRCA2 gene in my family, I'd want the test for it. You can make better decisions if you know."

---

38. *http://www.aarp.org/health/healthy-living/info-2014/sheryl-crow-melissa-etheridge-beat-cancer.html*

3-D Mammography

Three-dimensional (3-D) mammography, also known as breast tomosynthesis, is a type of digital mammography in which X-ray machines are used to take pictures of thin slices of the breast from different angles, and computer software is used to reconstruct an image. This process is similar to how a computed tomography (CT) scanner produces images of structures inside the body. Three-D mammography uses very low dose X-rays, but, because it is generally performed at the same time as standard two-dimensional (2-D) digital mammography, the radiation dose is slightly higher than that of standard mammography.

Since the accuracy of 3-D mammography has not been compared with that of 2-D mammography in randomized studies, researchers do not know whether 3-D mammography is better or worse than standard mammography at avoiding false-positive results and identifying early cancers.

MY JOURNEY

No one tipped me off that managing expectations would become one of the most challenging aspects of having cancer and dealing with the crazy assortment of tests, evaluations, and decisions I had to make, often on my own, it seemed, at crazy hours of the night when the only way I could get myself to sleep was by settling in on a course of action I could accept. For me, in times of unusual—and sometimes unbearable stress—I need people to be straight and give me the goods, even if it's bad. While a sugarcoated version may seem like a nice way to go, trust me, it's worthless. How can anyone make a serious choice if no one is leveling with them?

Kerry (Lincoln, Nebraska)

Cervical Cancer Screening

Regular screening of women between the ages of twenty-one and sixty-five years with a Pap test decreases their chance of dying from cervical cancer. In 1950, the Centers for Disease Control's (CDC) "Vital Statistics of the United States" reported an unadjusted death rate of 10.2 per 100,000 for white women and 18.0 for nonwhite women. By 2007, the age-adjusted mortality had dropped to 2.2 for white women, 4.3 for black women, and 2.4 overall.

Two main tests are used to screen for cervical cancer: the Papanicolaou (Pap) test and HPV test.

A Pap smear (also called a Pap test) is a procedure to collect cells from the surface of the cervix and vagina. A piece of cotton, a brush, or a small wooden stick is used to gently scrape cells that a pathologist views under a microscope to determine if they are abnormal.

The human papillomavirus (HPV) test is a laboratory measure used to check DNA or RNA for certain types of HPV infection. Cells collected from the cervix, including DNA or RNA from the cells, are checked to determine if an infection is caused by a type of HPV linked to cervical cancer.

This test may be done using a sample of cells removed during a Pap test. It may also be done if the results of a Pap test show certain abnormal cervical cells. When both the HPV test and Pap test are done using cells from the sample removed during a Pap test, it is called a Pap/HPV co-test.

Just as it is with mammography screening, the benefits of potential screening methods must be weighed against any potential harm caused by doing the test or reacting to the test results.

Benefits of Pap Screening

The rate at which invasive cancer develops from early dysplastic changes is usually slow, measured in years and possibly even decades.

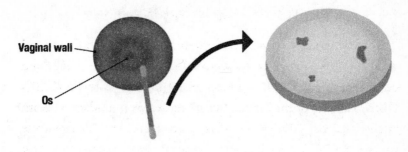

Pap Smear
Source: Joshua Abbas (*123rf.com*)

This long natural history provides the opportunity for screening to effectively detect this process during the preinvasive phase, thereby allowing for early treatment and a cure.

Although the Pap test has never been examined in a randomized controlled trial, a large body of consistent observational data supports its effectiveness in reducing mortality from cervical cancer. Both incidence and mortality from cervical cancer have sharply decreased in several large populations following the introduction of well-run screening programs.

But the news is not all positive.

Regular screening can lead to additional diagnostic procedures (such as colposcopy) and treatment for low-grade squamous intraepithelial lesions (LSIL), which can have long-term consequences for fertility and pregnancy. Younger women, who have a higher prevalence of LSIL, often have lesions that regress without treatment. The potential for harm also increases in younger women because they have a higher rate of false-positive results.

According to the National Cancer Institute, additional diagnostic procedures were performed in 50 percent of women undergoing regular Pap testing. Out of these, approximately 5 percent were treated for LSIL. The number with impaired fertility and pregnancy complications is unknown.

Liz Lange: Designer and Survivor

American fashion designer and entrepreneur Liz Lange is the founder of Liz Lange Maternity, which introduced form-fitting designer pregnancy wear in 1998. Business was really taking off by 2001 when her high-end maternity-wear line was all the rage with pregnant celebs like Kelly Ripa and Cindy Crawford.

When a routine pap smear at age thirty-five picked up cervical cancer, Liz didn't hesitate. She had two young children at home, Gus, then three, and Alice, one. She underwent a hysterectomy followed by radiation treatment and chemotherapy. Since then she has become an advocate for cervical cancer screening and a spokeswoman for the Gynecologic Cancer Foundation.

"As a survivor of cervical cancer," she told *The Huffington Post*, "I know just how fortunate I am to have beaten this disease. Like most women in the developed world, I had easy access to regular cervical-cancer screening, which caught my cancer early and ensured a positive long-term prognosis. My access to a regular Pap test ensured that I would not become one of the 270,000 women who die each year from cervical cancer."[39]

Pluses and Minuses of HPV Testing

Screening with HPV DNA or HPV RNA detects high-grade cervical dysplasia, a precursor lesion for cervical cancer. Additional clinical trials show that HPV testing is superior to other cervical cancer screening strategies. In April 2014, the U.S. Food and Drug Administration approved an HPV DNA test that can be used alone for the primary

---

39. *http://www.huffingtonpost.com/liz-lange/cervical-cancer-the-silent-killer-of-women-in-the-develop ing-world_b_1655231.html*

screening of cervical cancer risk in women aged twenty-five years and older.

HPV testing identifies numerous infections that will not lead to cervical dysplasia or cervical cancer. This is especially true in women younger than thirty, whose rates of HPV infection may be higher. In one study, 86.7 percent of women with a positive HPV test did not develop cervical cancer or related premalignant disease after more than a decade of follow-up.

Based on solid evidence from multiple experts, screening every five years with the Pap test and the HPV DNA test (co-testing) in women thirty years and older is more sensitive in detecting cervical abnormalities, compared with the Pap test, alone. However, co-testing is associated with more false-positives than just the Pap test. Abnormal test results can lead to more frequent testing and invasive diagnostic procedures.

Because cervical cancer is slow growing, considerable uncertainty surrounds the issue of the optimal screening interval. A large study that included data from the National Breast and Cervical Cancer Early Detection Program found little further mortality reduction from cervical cancer for screening every year as compared with screening every three years.

Current Guidelines for Cervical Cancer Screening in the United States

Having an annual Pap test to screen for early cervical cancer is no longer recommended by leading medical organizations, such as the American Cancer Society (ACS) and USPSTF.

Current recommendations are as follows:

- *No screening for women younger than twenty-one.* Cervical cancer is very rare in young women, and screening can lead to unnecessary follow-up tests or treatments, not to mention the emotional toll and psychological stress.

- *For women twenty-one to sixty-five years old,* a Pap smear should be done every three years *or* a Pap smear in combination with HPV testing every five years.
- *No screening for women over sixty-five* unless they are at high risk or lack prior screening data.

Endometrial Cancer Screening

Because endometrial cancer typically causes symptoms such as vaginal bleeding, it is often found at an early stage, when there is a good chance of recovery. At the current time, there is no standard or routine screening test for endometrial cancer. A few candidates have been evaluated and rejected for routine screening.

Transvaginal ultrasound (TVU) is a procedure used to examine the vagina, uterus, fallopian tubes, and bladder. An ultrasound probe is inserted into the vagina and used to bounce high-energy sound waves (ultrasound) off internal tissues or organs and make echoes. The echoes form a picture of body tissues called a sonogram. The doctor can identify tumors by looking at the sonogram.

Screening asymptomatic women with TVU will result in unnecessary additional biopsies because of false-positive test results. Risks associated with false-positive tests include anxiety and complications from biopsies.

Endometrial sampling is the removal of tissue from the endometrium by inserting a brush, curette, or thin, flexible tube through the cervix and into the uterus. The tool is used to gently scrape a small amount of tissue from the endometrium and then remove the tissue samples. A pathologist views the tissue under a microscope to look for cancer cells.

It has not been proven that a screening by endometrial sampling (biopsy) lowers the number of deaths caused by endometrial cancer.

Based on solid evidence, endometrial biopsy may result in discomfort, bleeding, infection, and, rarely, uterine perforation.

Ovarian Cancer Screening

Perhaps one of the most frustrating failures for women's cancer screening is found in ovarian cancer screening. Ovarian cancer often presents itself with persistent, vague symptoms, and usually occurs after the cancer has already metastasized. Even a manual pelvic exam, part of a routine pelvic examination, can detect only advanced disease.

Transvaginal ultrasound (TVU) has been investigated as a screening method for ovarian cancer. Although TVU is fairly reliable in measuring ovarian size and detecting small masses, solid evidence indicates that screening for ovarian cancer with TVU does not result in a decrease in ovarian cancer mortality, even after an average follow-up of over twelve years.

CA-125 is a tumor-associated antigen that is used clinically to monitor patients with epithelial ovarian carcinomas. Measurement of CA-125 concentrations has been proposed as a potential marker for the early detection of ovarian cancer, either as a single test with a threshold cutoff point or in watching the change in levels over time. Once again, the results have been less than promising. Elevated CA-125 levels are not specific to ovarian cancer and have been observed in patients with many other conditions, including non-gynecological cancers, fluid accumulation in the pleura (lung cavity) or peritoneum (abdominal cavity), in early pregnancy, or in women with endometriosis.

The test wasn't particularly sensitive, either. A 2011 study[40] detected only eleven of nineteen cases of ovarian cancer using CA-125 levels.

False-positive test results can have serious consequences. Screened

---

40. *http://www.ncbi.nlm.nih.gov/pubmed/8490497?dopt=Abstract*

women had higher rates of oophorectomy (removal of the ovaries) as well as other minor complications, such as fainting and bruising.

Several biomarkers with potential application to ovarian cancer screening are under development but have not yet been validated or evaluated for efficacy in early detection and mortality reduction.

─────────────── **MY JOURNEY** ───────────────

As I progress through treatment, which includes a perpetual round of tests and scans and more scans and tests, balancing fear and hope is an ongoing struggle, sometimes even more than whatever physical discomfort I may be going through. Sometimes, I think I may be afraid to hope, especially if a scan comes back with good news. I mean, what if the next one doesn't? Can I relax for the next month or three or six until the next one? Living in the moment is my new challenge. I always thought that a phrase like that contained a simple idea. Live in the moment—what can be so hard about that? But over the course of the last few years, as I have endured more and more rounds of treatment and testing, I have come to realize that this type of existence—living from scan to scan—is the hardest part of this whole ordeal. So now, almost seven years later, I don't think about cancer every day, but my positive and negative sides still exist in a virtual tug-of-war, and God only knows who is winning.

Marcia (Baltimore, Maryland)

Where Do We Go from Here?

Centers for Disease Control statistics show that in the 1930s, uterine and cervical cancers were the leading causes of cancer deaths among American women. In the 1950s, when using the Pap test began in earnest, rates of death from cervical cancer declined significantly. With the continued development of a variety of new testing to detect the presence of cancer through imaging procedures, death rates *and* the number of women getting the disease in the first place are continuing to drop.

But at the same time, several studies predict that the frequency of breast cancer cases in the United States will increase more than 50 percent in the coming decades, which is largely due to an aging population.

A new study led by Philip Rosenberg, PhD, of NCI's Division of Cancer Epidemiology and Genetics and presented at the AACR annual meeting last year, acknowledged this increase but predicted proportionately fewer cases considered difficult regarding treatment.

Meanwhile, as efforts continue to make women's cancer screening available to everyone, especially those in underserved communities, we can take heart that the numbers are generally improving—some at a faster rate than was imagined just a few years ago.

It takes a village—patient, provider, and healthcare system—working together to make effective cancer screening programs that can achieve high screening rates. It's a question of synergy, combining better patient responsibility, innovations in technology, increased access to primary care services, community organizing, and improvements in the insurance system to create an environment that can better serve the needs of America's women and their families. There are lessons to be learned about screening programs from success stories in this country and around the world. Now is the time to urge our political and business leaders to prioritize these improvements.

KEY POINTS TO REMEMBER

✓ At its root, cancer is a disease of your DNA.

✓ Knowing your family medical history, screening, and early detection will be the main tools for saving your life from cancer.

✓ It is important to note the potential risks regarding screening tests.

✓ Early detection is vital. When cancer is found early, it is almost always easier to treat.

✓ Most cancers are not caused by inherited genes but by damage to your DNA that occurs in your lifetime.

✓ Chemoprevention refers to the use of drugs to lower the risk of cancer or its recurrence.

✓ Contrary to popular claims, vitamin and dietary supplements have not been shown to prevent cancer.

✓ Aspirin is being studied for the prevention of invasive ovarian cancer and breast cancer, as well as for colorectal cancer.

✓ Although mammograms can detect malignant tumors that cannot be felt during an external breast exam, treating a small tumor does not always mean that a woman's life will be saved.

✓ Having an annual Pap test to screen for early cervical cancer is no longer recommended by leading medical organizations.

✓ Because endometrial cancer typically causes symptoms such as vaginal bleeding, it is often found at an early stage, when there is a good chance of recovery.

My Revelation

As I spiral deeper into my treatments,
Sometimes I have the feeling I am sleeping next to myself.
It's calming, almost, until I notice I am drifting away,
Losing my center and what has always grounded me.
Scared, yes, but I keep my pilot light going.

I am slowing down, growing more quiet, vanishing into survival mode,
Knowing I am confused, that I can't always feel the steps beneath my feet.
I am floating somewhere, somewhere I've never been before.
Will I find myself again?
Maybe yes, maybe no . . . but at least it's me who's looking.

—Daniela Palik

14 EMBRACING THE TWENTY-FIRST CENTURY: Changing Definitions and the Future of Cancer

Cancer affects all of us, whether you're a daughter, mother, sister, friend, coworker, doctor, or patient.

—Jennifer Aniston, actress

A Wake-Up Call

On the evening of August 27, 2013, approximately 32,000 American women went to sleep thinking they had been diagnosed with breast cancer. When they woke up the next morning, their cancer was gone. Was it some kind of miracle or act of God? Neither one, in fact, because as the sun rose the next day, a group of medical experts concluded that the disease these women had could no longer be called "cancer" at all.

These experts were talking about DCIS of the breast, a condition that will *never* become invasive cancer in 70 to 80 percent of women with this diagnosis (Chapter 2). In the past, about 98 percent of women with this "stage 0 cancer" would undergo invasive treatments for this disease, such as lumpectomy, radiation therapy, or mastectomy—at great cost as well as emotional and physical distress. In the future, most of these women will probably be treated with what is called "watchful waiting."

The prominent breast surgeon Dr. Laura Esserman of the Diller Family Cancer Center at the University of California at San Francisco (UCSF) has recommended changing the name of DCIS to IDLE (indolent lesions of epithelial origin). This change not only describes the condition more accurately but also eliminates the specter of cancer from the diagnosis.

In Chapter 6, we explained how decades of medical dogma about ovarian cancer now must be reimagined and revised because this silent killer of women actually arises in the fallopian tubes and is now called pelvic serous carcinoma (PSC).

In the future, so-called ovarian cancer may be prevented by simply removing a woman's fallopian tubes after her childbearing years, or earlier, if she's genetically at risk.

This situation has been nicely summarized by the Chief Medical Officer of the American Cancer Society, Dr. Otis Brawley, who has said, "We need a twenty-first-century definition of cancer instead of a nineteenth-century definition, which is what we've been using."

After decades of research, scientists now understand that cancer is not one singular disease but hundreds of different diseases, all of which result from "misprints" (mutations) in our DNA. These diseases affect everyone differently. In fact, not all of the conditions we traditionally refer to as cancer will inexorably progress to metastases and death. For an increasing number of cancers, they will be viewed as simply another chronic illness, like type 2 diabetes or high blood pressure. Treatments will be designed to manage the cancer instead of always trying to destroy it with harsh methods that have serious side effects. Treatment will be based on precision diagnosis and personalized treatment for each unique patient.

Reimagining Diagnosis and Treatment

In the not-too-distant future, a blood test to detect many types of cancer may just be another part of your annual physical, like checking your blood sugar and cholesterol. Researchers have recently discovered that once cancer forms, even if it's too small to see on an X-ray or CT scan, some cancer cells break down and leak their tumor DNA into the bloodstream.

There is abundant research currently studying whether liquid biopsies (blood tests) to detect this "circulating tumor DNA" (ctDNA) can be used for early detection of cancer, monitoring treatment responses, and early detection of recurrences or resistance to treatments.

Technologically, it's getting easier and cheaper all the time to check large collections of genes for smoking gun mutations that indicate cancer, even for the very tiny amounts of ctDNA that tumors leak into the bloodstream.

What could this mean for patients?

In Chapter 6, we reported that mutations in a gene called TP53 seem to be early events in the development of ovarian (pelvic serous) cancer. What if future research shows that we can detect abnormal copies of TP53 DNA leaked into the blood by these early cancers? Would such a test be run every year on high-risk women like BRCA1 and BRAC2 carriers who could use this information to help them decide when or if to undergo prophylactic surgery? Could such a test even be used in all women, with the goal of catching early cancers years before they grow out of control and start producing symptoms?

Another recent advance is the development of immunotherapy drugs that attack cancer cells in an entirely different way than drugs targeted at specific cancer genes. In some cancers, such as malignant melanoma and lung cancer, tumor cells are known to harbor a plethora of abnormal changes in their DNA, called a high mutational burden.

To make a long story short, these numerous DNA defects can lead to changes in the cells that make them look like foreign invaders in our immune systems. But cancer cells are devious and usually find ways to escape an immune response. The new drugs called immune checkpoint inhibitors block the cancer from escaping and enable special immune cells, T-cells, to capture and kill the tumor.

Four of these new drugs are currently available, and one was used in the near-miraculous cure of former President Jimmy Carter, whose malignant skin cancer (melanoma) had invaded both his liver and brain. Immune checkpoint inhibitors currently approved by the FDA to treat cancer include:

- Ipilimumab (Yervoy), approved to treat advanced melanoma (skin cancer)
- Nivolumab (Opdivo), approved to treat advanced melanoma, some types of lung cancer, and kidney cancer
- Pembrolizumab (Keytruda), approved to treat advanced melanoma and some types of lung cancer
- Atezolizumab (Tecentriq), to treat advanced bladder cancer after other treatments have failed

In fact, this "immune checkpoint" approach to treating cancer is so promising that pharmaceutical companies are investing large amounts of money and research into developing more drugs of this type. They are also testing in clinical research trials how these existing drugs can be used to treat more types of cancer, including breast cancer (Chapter 2).

──── MY JOURNEY ────

I am not a doctor. I do not have cancer. But I am sure that love can help to cure it. Excuse me that I cannot produce any scientific evidence for this, but I have seen it work when my mother was diagnosed. At first, everyone in our house was silent, as if we might say the wrong thing simply by opening our mouths. Then I saw my father so tenderly holding my mother's hand and my sister stroking her hair. As I watched, I could not only see the smile emerging on my mother's face. I could feel her healing right in front of me! I knew in that moment that her cure could not come only from her doctors and the treatments they prescribed. It was up to us, and her, to coax away the cancer with love—with a fierce, unbending song of positivity.

That's what we did. We eliminated any shred of negativity from our house and replaced it with love, every minute of every day. Every painful moment my mother felt was accompanied by a loving touch, a terrible joke, and a soothing bit of music. Every moment of fear was met with a lovely dream to look forward to. This became our normal way to live, and when my mother was supposed to feel sick from treatment, she began to stabilize. When her doctors expected her to suffer, she did not. All the love penetrated every one of her cells, until she began to love herself in ways I had never before witnessed. I believe this gave her strength and a resolve she may not have had before, and this carried her, too, along with our love.

Now, a few years later, my mother is cancer-free and volunteering at the center, encouraging patients and doctors and nurses, anyone she comes into contact with, to embrace the power of love. I am no doctor, but I do know that love can do magic. It can even cure cancer.

Jamie (Hartford, Connecticut)

Do We Need a "Moonshot" to Cure Cancer?
And Why Now?

In President Obama's January 2016 State of the Union address, he called for a new "moonshot" to cure cancer—a program to be led by Vice President Joe Biden, whose son Beau died of brain cancer in May 2015. "This is personal for me," Biden told *AARP The Magazine* in March 2016. "But this is personal for just about every American and millions around the world."

As we've explained throughout this book, tremendous advances have been made in cancer research and treatment since 2001. In fact, during these past fifteen years, so many advances have accumulated that we have now reached a critical mass of knowledge and experience, placing us on the brink of transforming cancer into a manageable illness, even if we might not be able to completely cure it in all cases.

This accumulated knowledge base is a launching pad for an attack on cancer so broad and meaningful that nothing like it has been seen since President Nixon first declared the War on Cancer forty-five years ago, in 1971.

Specific plans for this concentrated push to cure cancer are still being drawn up as we complete this book, but allow us to share our vision of what we would like the goals of this cancer moonshot to be.

Goal #1: Better Education and New Tools for Training Healthcare Professionals

Advances in cancer diagnosis and treatment have been so rapid that most doctors never learn about them in medical school. The result is that even currently available drugs and diagnostics are being underutilized or improperly utilized. According to a March 2015 story in *Time*, fewer than 5 percent of the 1.6 million people diagnosed with cancer each year in the United States have access to cancer DNA testing. One important reason is that many doctors don't understand the technology and how best to use it.

The March 2013 issue of *O, The Oprah Magazine*, said, "DNA research has led to cutting-edge breakthroughs in how we detect cancer risk. But when doctors can't keep up with the science, the results can be perilous."

As the *New York Times* reported earlier this year, "The genetic data is there, but in many cases, doctors do not know what to do with it."[41]

Goal #2: Applied Research in the Optimal Use of Currently Available Therapies

At the present time, about sixty targeted drugs and immunotherapies have been approved by the FDA for the treatment of various types of cancer. Traditionally, a new cancer drug is approved to treat only one type of cancer but is later found to be useful for other cancer types, based on underlying genetic similarities among diverse tumor types. Remember imatinib (Gleevec) from Chapter 1? This drug was originally approved (indicated) in 2001 to treat one relatively uncommon blood cancer called CML. But now, fifteen years later, the indications of imatinib have expanded to at least eight different types of cancers or cancer-like conditions.

Another example is how and when to use individual drugs or combinations and how to sequence these therapies at different times. For example, melanoma could be successfully treated with a single drug (monotherapy) called vemurafenib (Zelboraf), but most patients developed resistance to treatment and their cancers came back after a year. Doctors discovered that combination therapy with two different drugs (dabrafenib [Tafinlar] and trametinib [Mekinist]), which attack

---

41. Gina Kolata, "When Gene Tests for Breast Cancer Reveal Grim Data but No Guidance," *New York Times*, March 11, 2016.

different weak points in the tumor at the same time, leads to more durable responses—meaning the tumors don't come back as quickly, or at all. Things are changing once again in the treatment of melanoma patients, with many doctors treating first with immunotherapies and saving the gene-targeted drugs to be used later, if necessary.

Goal #3: Development of New Services Unique to Long-Term Survivors

If many cancers really do become manageable chronic illnesses, like high blood pressure or diabetes, patients will need new types of services and resources to help with special challenges, such as coping with side effects or aftereffects of treatment. In Chapters 5 and 11, we describe two new medical specialties, oncoplastic surgery and onco-cardiology, that have recently arisen in response to new needs of patients.

Goal #4: Pursuit of New Biomedical Research Opportunities

In the May 19, 2016, issue of *The New England Journal of Medicine*, Dr. Douglas Lowy, Director of the National Cancer Institute, and Dr. Francis Collins, Director of the National Institutes of Health, published a plan for the Cancer Moonshot Program. It promised that by the end of the summer of 2016, a Blue Ribbon Panel would provide recommendations to the National Cancer Advisory Board on the most exceptional opportunities in cancer research. These are likely to include early detection technologies, cancer vaccines and immunotherapies, unique aspects of childhood cancers, and data sharing intended to break down barriers between public and private research organizations.

Challenges for Patients and Society

We must mention one fundamental factor that needs to be a priority of President Obama's moonshot. In fact, it may be the only way that any of these potential advances can come to fruition, saving millions of people from suffering unnecessarily from cancer.

That is the study of onco-economics—the economics of cancer care.

All of the exciting developments that we've talked about create formidable economic challenges for society. The first reason is that patients will live much longer but require treatment and new services for the rest of their lives. Second, a single targeted cancer drug or immunotherapy can cost thousands of dollars per month. If a new standard of care involves combinations of drugs that have to be taken for years, the potential costs become staggering.

Together, we all need to figure out the best ways to tackle cancer and save our own lives. As we've mentioned repeatedly, prevention needs to come first and that is a team effort that needs all of us to participate.

KEY POINTS TO REMEMBER

✓ We need a twenty-first-century definition of cancer instead of a nineteenth-century definition.

✓ During the past fifteen years, so many advances have been made that we have now reached a critical mass of knowledge and experience that allows us to reimagine cancer as a manageable illness.

✓ Some diseases we used to call cancer have been "downgraded" with less frightening names.

✓ Some cancer treatments are being de-intensified.

✓ In the not-too-distant future, a blood test to detect many types of cancer may just be another part of your annual physical exam.

✓ In the future, so-called ovarian cancer may be prevented by simply removing a woman's fallopian tubes after her childbearing years, or earlier if she's genetically at risk.

✓ Onco-economics refers to the economics of cancer care.

✓ Prevention needs to come first, and that is a team effort that needs all of us to participate.

HOPE IS UNDEFEATED

Blood counts soar and drop,
Skin goes raw and teeth fall out,
Hair, what hair, it's everywhere but on my head.

I can't walk much without a rest,
My dinner tastes like cardboard,
If they poke another vein, I might explode.

The prognosis, the psychosis,
It's just a phase of my neurosis,
Oh my, I can't keep up with all the talk.

I have what I need to keep going,
Nothing else matters, even in the dark,
Because it's mine, it's mine to have and hold.

No matter what the scan is saying,
In spite of all I suffer well,
Nothing can really touch me.

My hope goes undefeated.

—Anonymous

About the Authors

Michele R. Berman, MD

Michele Berman, MD, is a graduate of Washington University School of Medicine in St. Louis, Missouri, and completed her residency in Pediatrics at Children's Hospital in St. Louis. She served as Staff Pediatrician at DePaul Hospital in Bridgeton, Missouri, and as Clinical Instructor at Georgetown University and George Washington University in Washington, DC. She practiced general pediatrics in a private practice on Capitol Hill for twelve years. She also served on courtesy or active staff at other Washington area medical facilities, including Children's Hospital National Medical Center, Columbia Hospital for Women, Holy Cross Hospital, and Shady Grove Adventist Hospital.

During her sixteen years in primary care medical practice, Dr. Berman interacted with thousands of "consumers," explaining to them complex medical concepts in layperson's terms. This experience was supplemented and extended through her monthly consumer advice column in *Washington Parent Magazine*.

In 1997, she established one of the first private practice websites in the country—*ThePediatricCenter.com*—in Washington, DC, and Bethesda, Maryland. This site served as an additional communication channel for the consumer health information in her *Washington Parent* articles, and it employed rudimentary social networking features such as patients submitting their school artwork to be featured on the site.

In late 2008, Dr. Berman founded Celebrity Diagnosis to take her medical journalism to Web 2.0 communications. This work has been recognized by several local and national media organizations, such as the *Wall Street Journal*, the *Boston Globe*, Fox25 News, and WCVB News in Boston, New England Cable News, and the *San Diego Union-Tribune*. Since January 2009, she has written 200 stories about cancer and has written or coauthored over 1,000 articles about other diseases, medical conditions, and consumer health topics.

Many people follow her tweets on Twitter and posts on Facebook, including consumers, physicians, nurses, psychologists, nutritionists, medical writers, social media marketing experts, women's magazines, the Pew Internet and American Life Project, the Robert Wood Johnson Foundation, the Medicine and Health editor for *USA Today* (Liz Szabo), and *American Medical News*.

Dr. Berman is a Fellow of the American Academy of Pediatrics, a former Member of the Medical Society of the District of Columbia, and the Montgomery County Medical Society. Her awards include Phi Beta Kappa from Johns Hopkins University and Omicron Delta Kappa from Johns Hopkins University's National Leadership Society.

HealthPlus Health Plan named her Outstanding Primary Care Physician, and she has been cited by *Washingtonian Magazine* as an Outstanding Washington Physician.

Mark S. Boguski, MD, PhD, FCAP

D r. **Mark S. Boguski** is the founder and Chief Medical Officer of Precision Medicine Network, Inc.

He has served on the faculties at Harvard Medical School and Beth Israel Deaconess Medical Center, the Johns Hopkins University School of Medicine, the Fred Hutchinson Cancer Research Center, and the National Institutes of Health. He is a former faculty member of the Molecular Biology in Clinical Oncology workshop at the American Association for Cancer Research.

Dr. Boguski has also served as Vice President of the Novartis Institute for Biomedical Research and as the founding Director of the Paul Allen Institute for Brain Science. He has been an advisor and consultant to numerous medical research organizations, including the Merck Genome Research Institute, the Genetics Advisory Group for the Welcome Trust, and the Howard Hughes Medical Institute.

Dr. Boguski has received the Regents' Award from the National Library of Medicine and the Director's Award from the National Institutes of Health. He is an elected member of the US National Academy of Medicine, a Fellow of the College of American Pathologists, and a Fellow of the

American College of Medical Informatics, as well as former reviewing editor for *Science* magazine and past editor in chief of the journal *Genomics*.

Dr. Boguski received his BA from The Johns Hopkins University and an MD and PhD from the Medical Scientist Training Program at the Washington University School of Medicine.

David Tabatsky

David Tabatsky is a writer, editor, teacher, director, and performing artist. He received his BA in Communications and an MA in Theatre Education, both from Adelphi University.

David is the author of *Write for Life: Communicating Your Way Through Cancer* and coauthor of *The Cancer Book: 101 Stories of Courage, Support and Love*, and editor of Elizabeth Bayer's *It's Just a Word*, the last two published by Chicken Soup for the Soul Publishing in 2009. He is the coauthor with Bruce Kluger of *Dear President Obama: Letters of Hope from Children Across America*, also published in 2009. David wrote *The Boy Behind the Door: How Salomon Kool Escaped the Nazis* (2009). With Dr. Mark Banschick, David coauthored *The Intelligent Divorce*—Books One and Two (2009 and 2010, respectively)—and *The Wright Choice: Your Family's Guide to Healthy Eating, Modern Fitness and Saving Money* (2011) with Dr. Randy Wright. David was the consulting editor for Marlo Thomas and her *New York Times* bestseller *The Right Words at the Right Time, Volume 2: Your Turn* (2006). He has published two editions of *What's Cool Berlin*, a comic travel guide to Germany's capital, and has written for *The Forward, Parenting,* and *Sesame Street Parent,* among others.

David has worked professionally in theater and circus as an actor, clown, and juggler at New York City's Lincoln Center, Radio City Music Hall, the Beacon Theatre, and throughout the United States and Europe, most notably at the Chamäleon in Berlin, New End Theatre in London, Folies Pigalle in Paris, and the Edinburgh Fringe Festival, where *THE STAGE* wrote, "He is a supremely skillful performer and a fine actor, reaching levels no other comics have matched at this Fringe." David also directed Kinderzirkus Taborka at the renowned Tempodrom in Berlin.

David has taught theater and circus arts for the American School of

London, die Etage in Berlin, the Big Apple Circus School, The United Nations International School, and the Cathedral of St. John the Divine. He served on the theater faculty at Adelphi University and The Cooper Union, and as a teaching artist for The Henry Street Settlement, with a focus on special education. He has taught circus arts at Sunrise Day Camp, America's only dedicated day camp for children with cancer and their siblings.

David teaches writing and communication workshops and speaks on these subjects at cancer centers throughout the United States.

Please visit *www.tabatsky.com* and *www.writeforlife.info*.

About *Reimagining Men's Cancers*

America's fascination with celebrities never gets old and their stories can educate people about important issues, including cancer. In fact, they can save a life.

That's what *Reimagining Men's Cancers* exemplifies by focusing on cancers of the prostate, penis, breast, and testicles—providing readers with critical information about basic anatomy diagnosis, scientific guidelines and a survey of treatments and prevention.

Woven throughout are celebrity stories, from men such as Joe Torre, Robert De Niro, and Kareem Abdul-Jabbar, as well as from "normal" people you may recognize as your friends, colleagues, and family members.

See more at *http://www.hcibooks.com/p-4381-reimagining-mens -cancers.aspx#sthash.9XifoVaF.dpuf*.

Index